Coffee, Scrubs and Rubber Gloves A Coloring Book for Nurses

Hi everyone,

Thank you so much for purchasing this coloring book. I hope you enjoy it!

I have a special surprise for you…

Claim your gift here: https://bit.ly/2K58AtH

Thanks so much and happy coloring!

Color Test Page

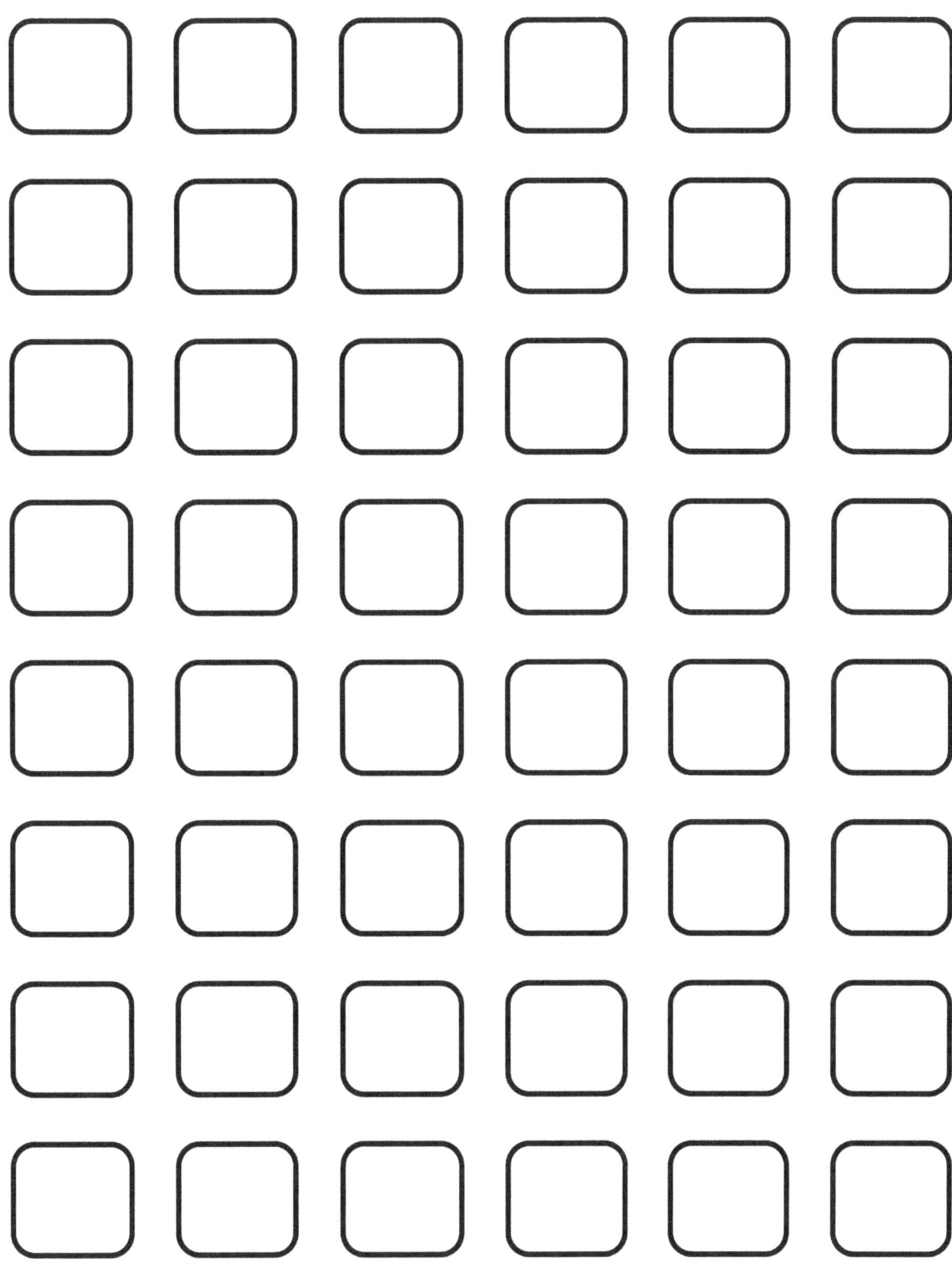

Color Test Page

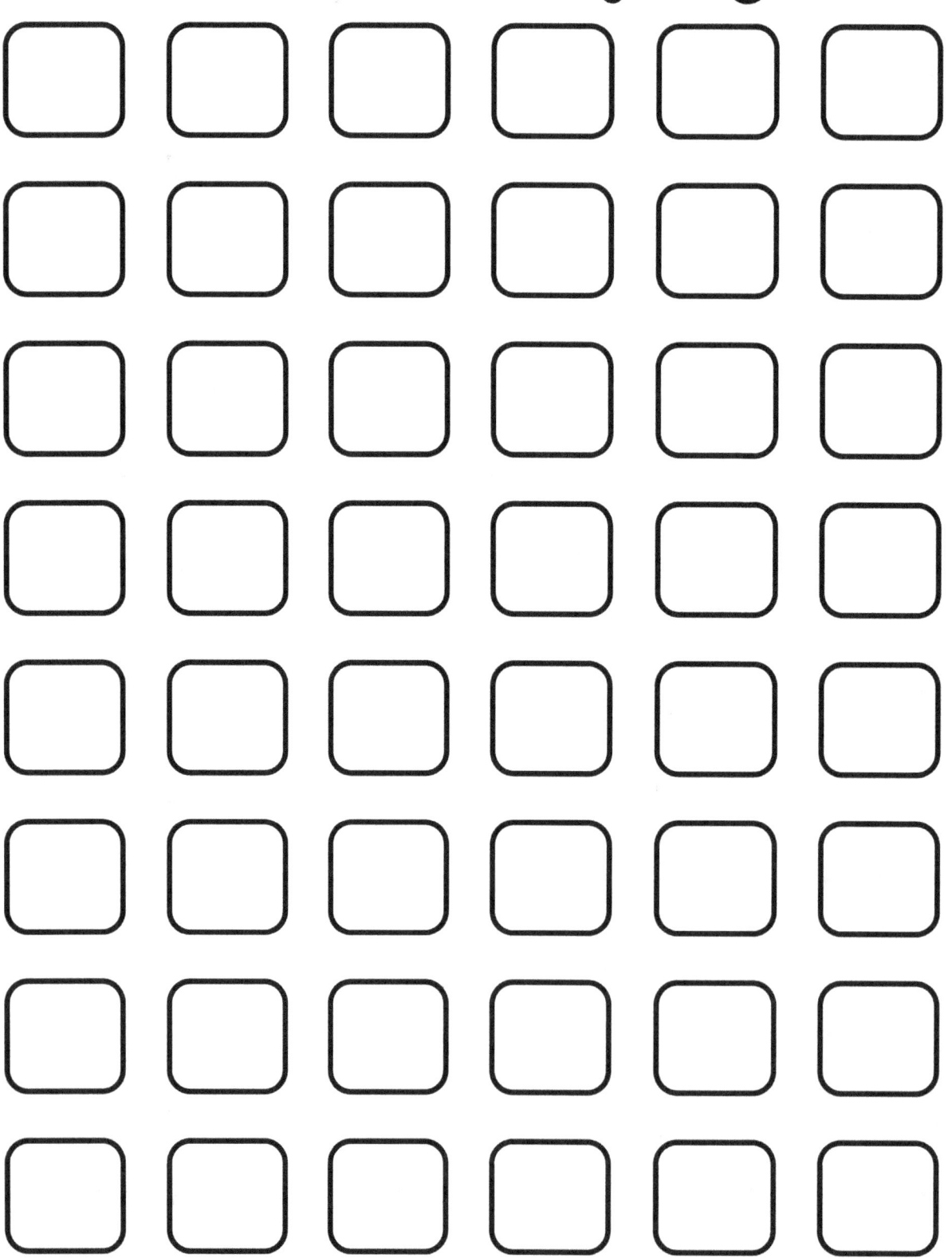

I'm just taking your vital signs

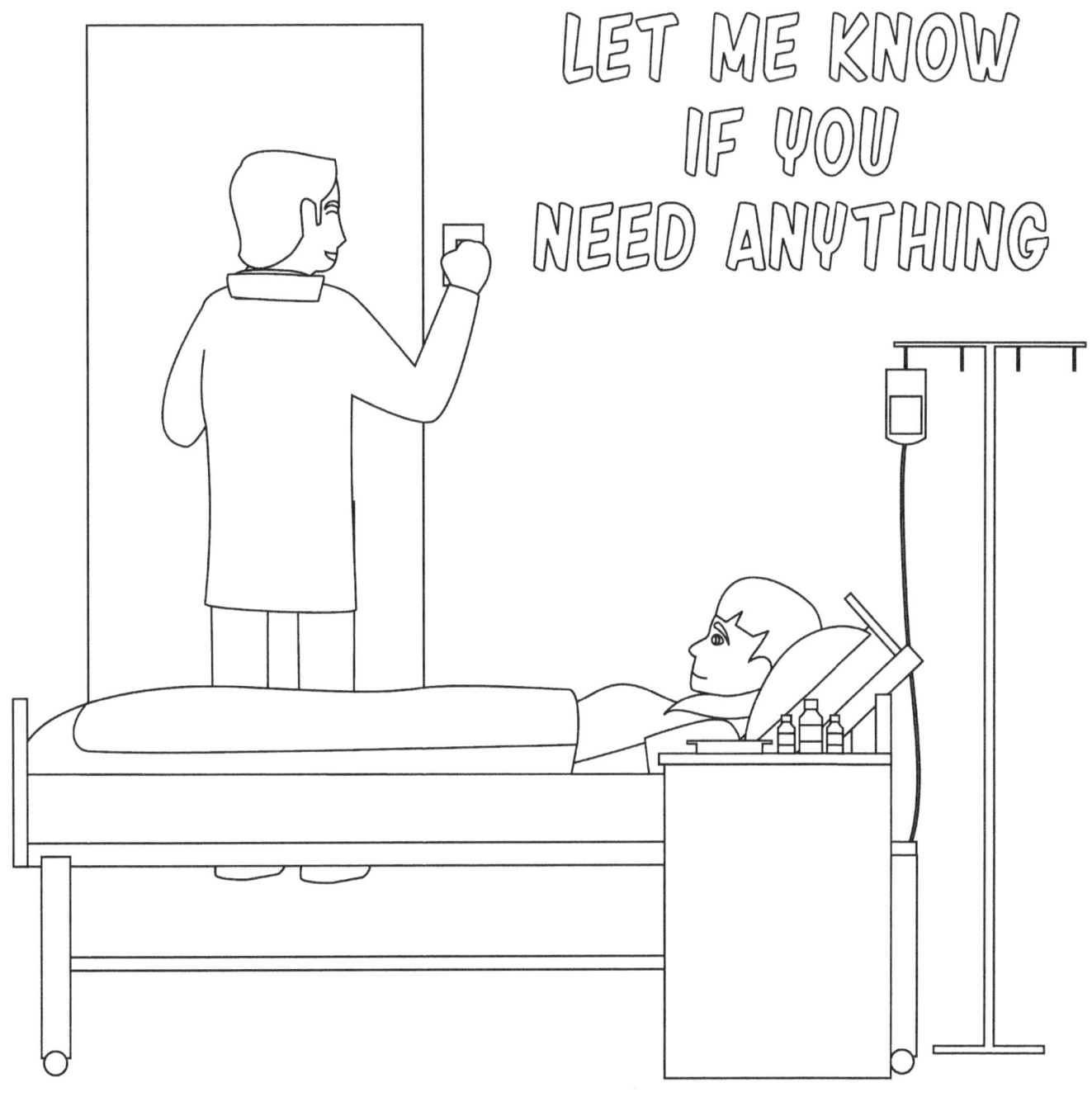

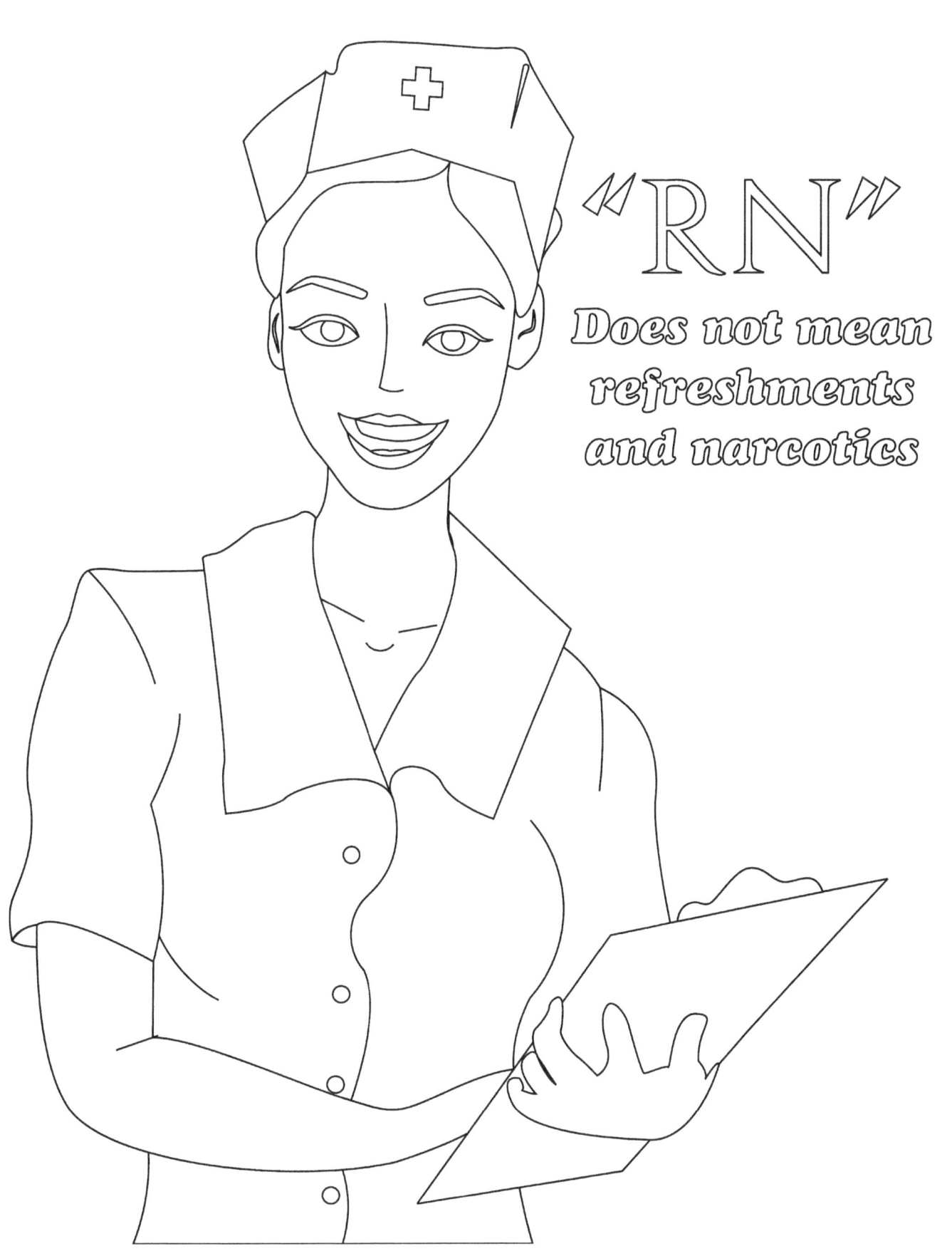

I'VE GOT DESIGNER

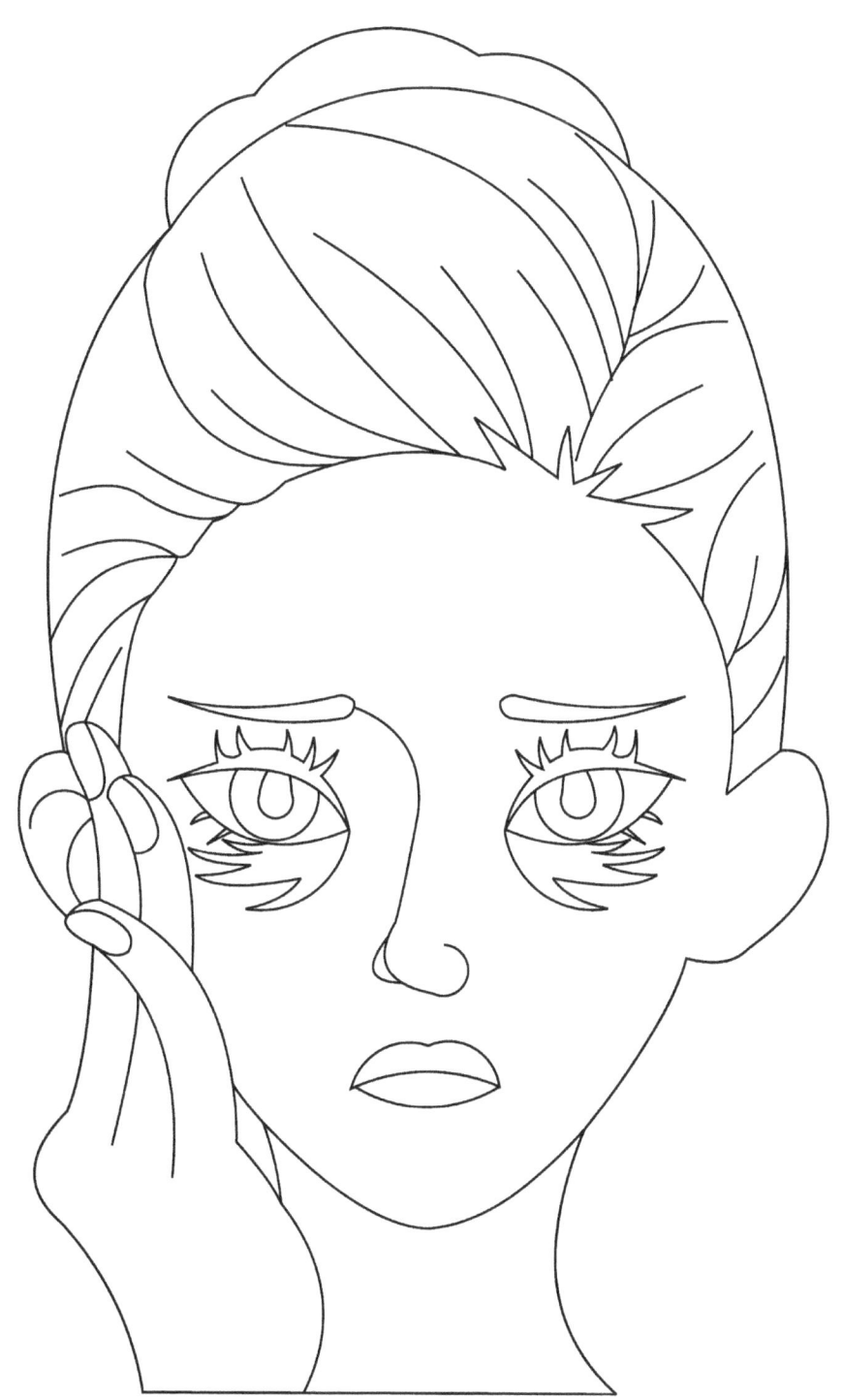

BAGS UNDER MY EYES

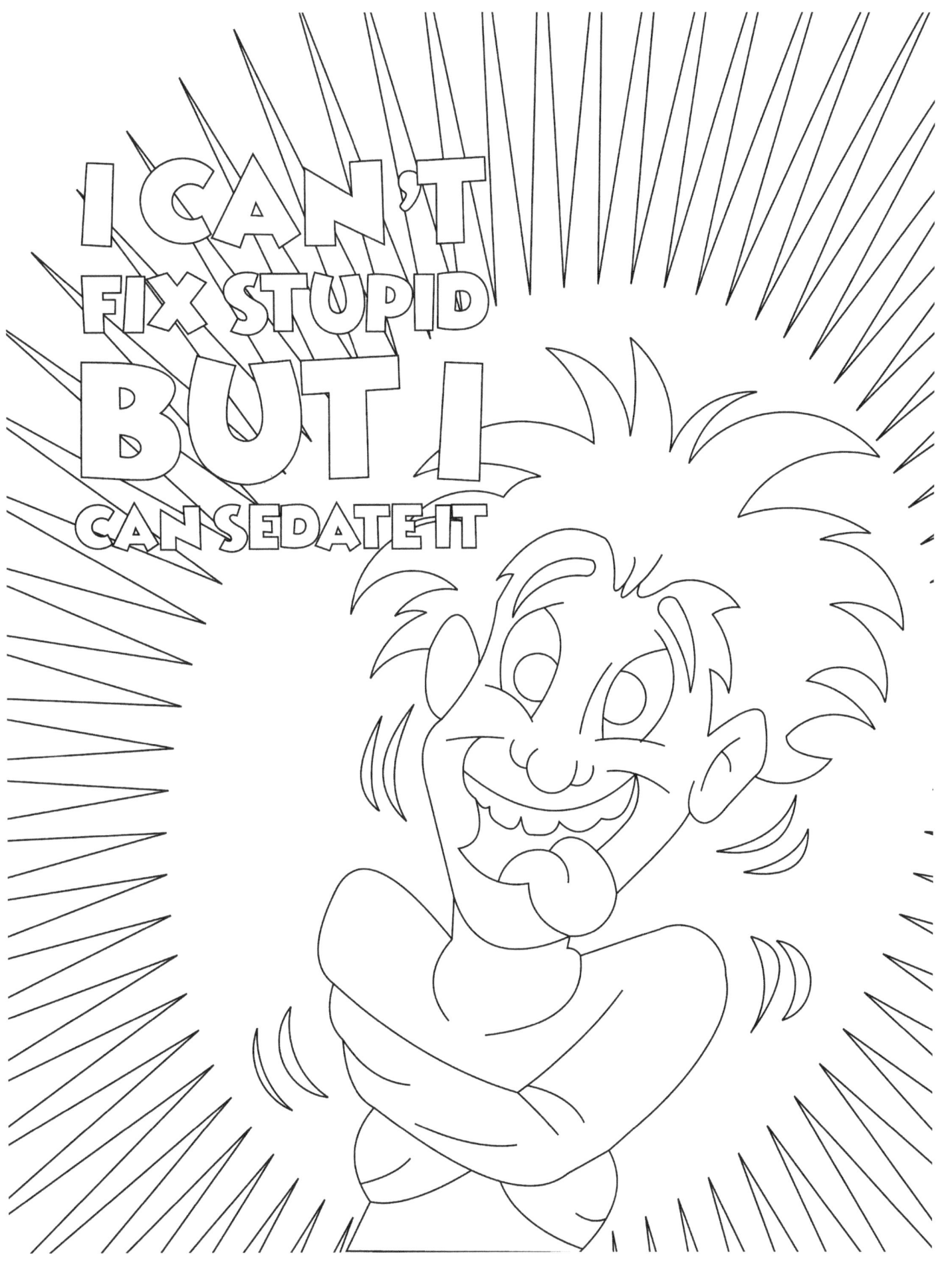

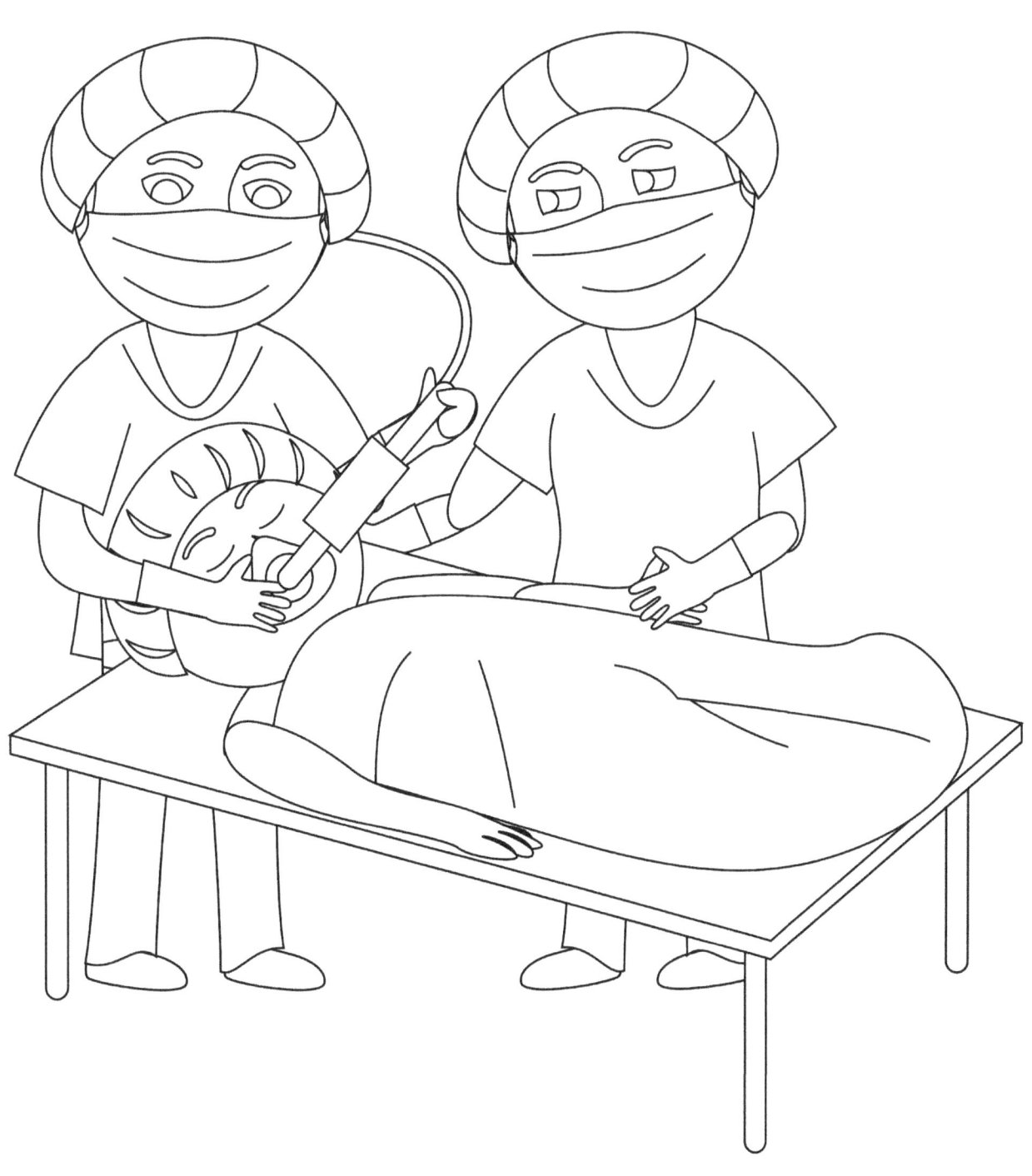

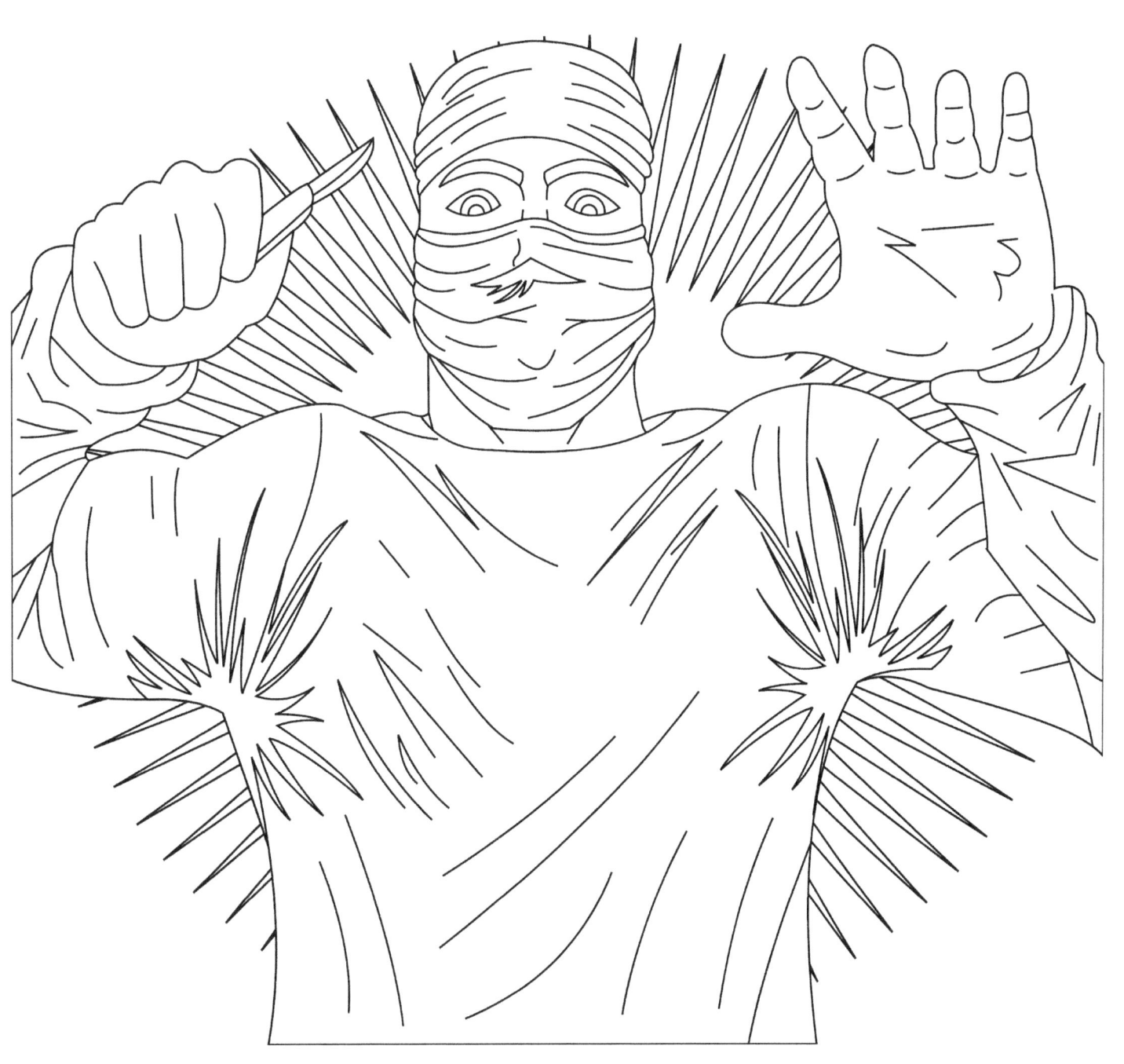

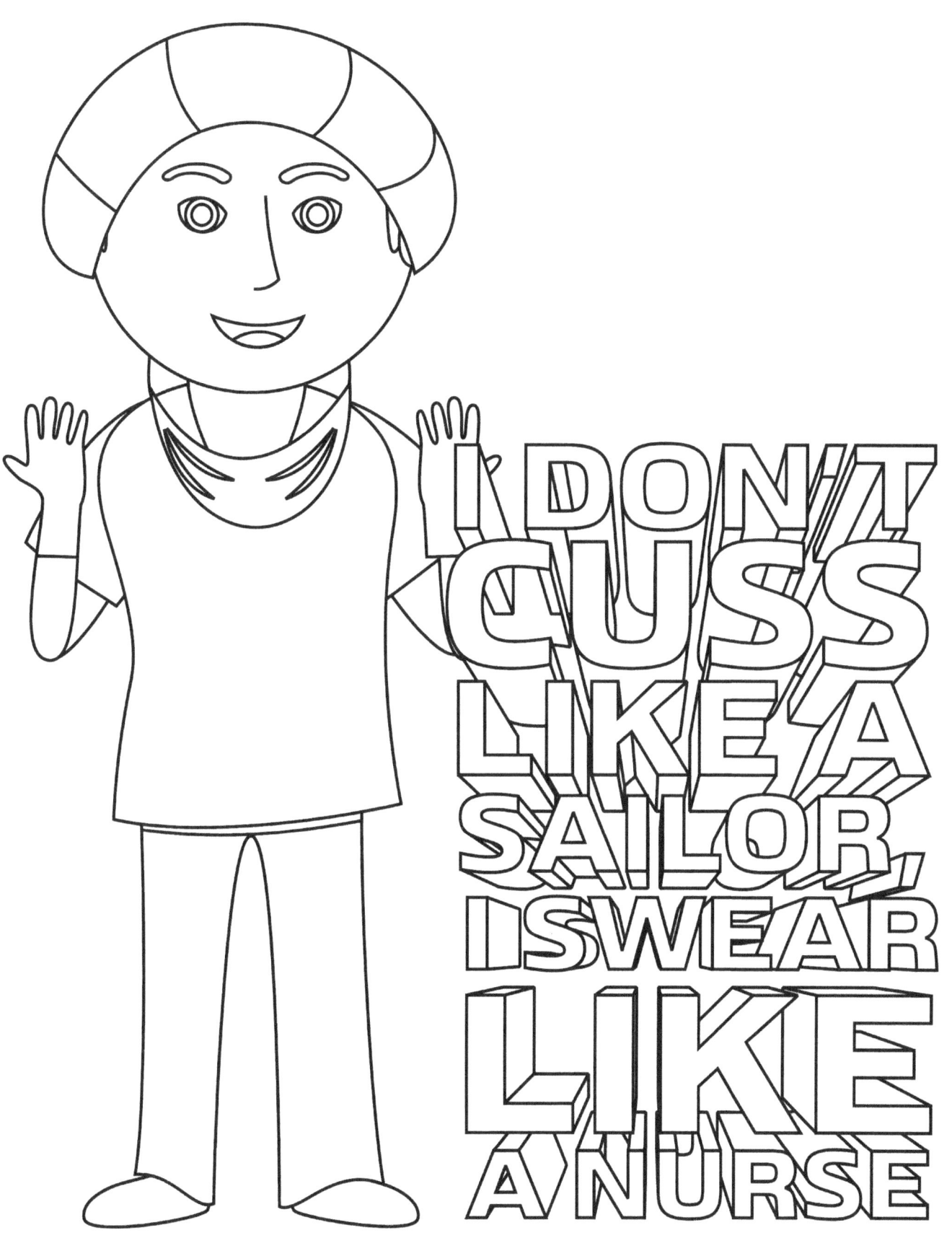

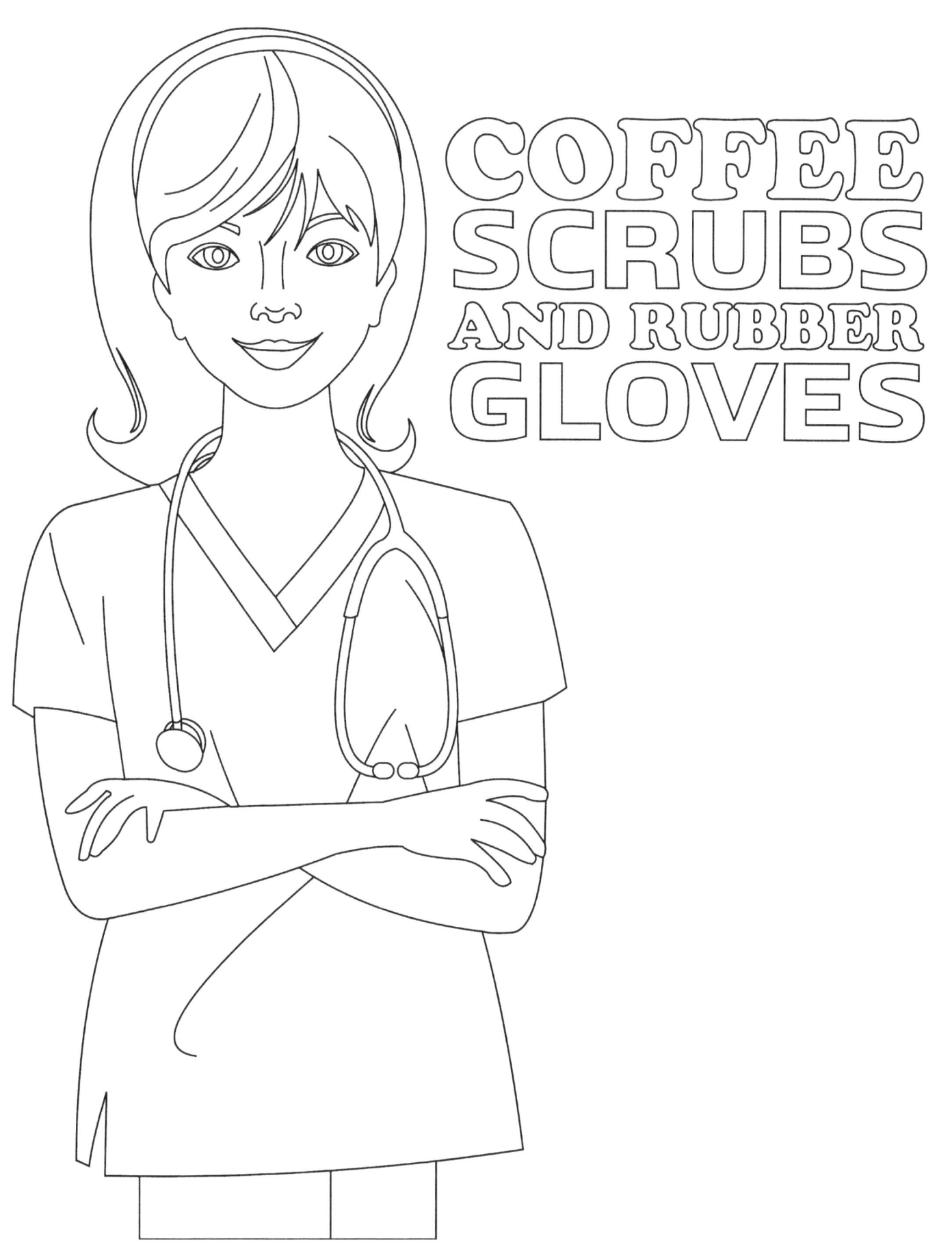

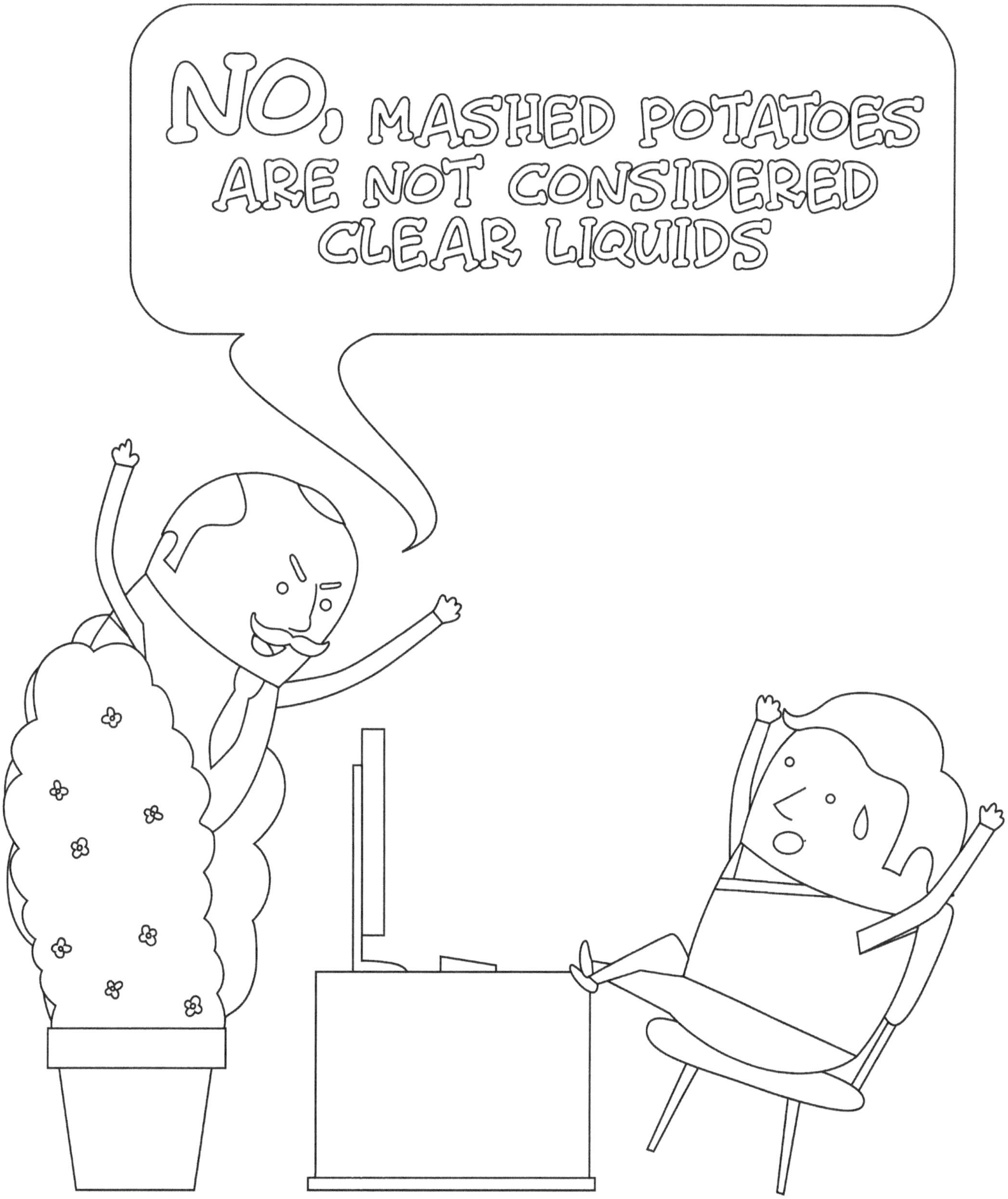

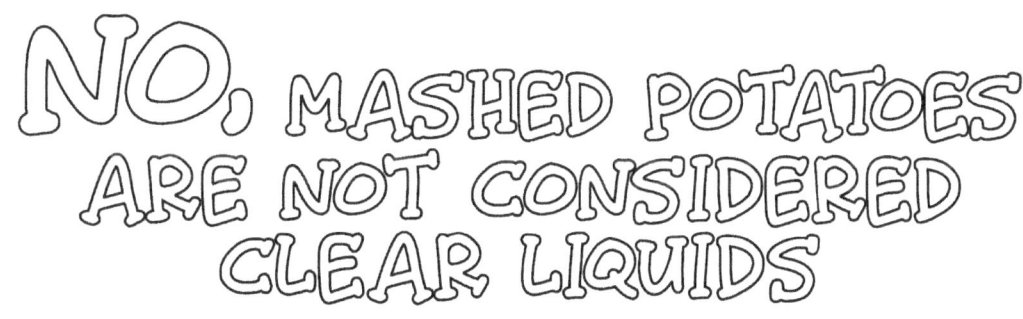

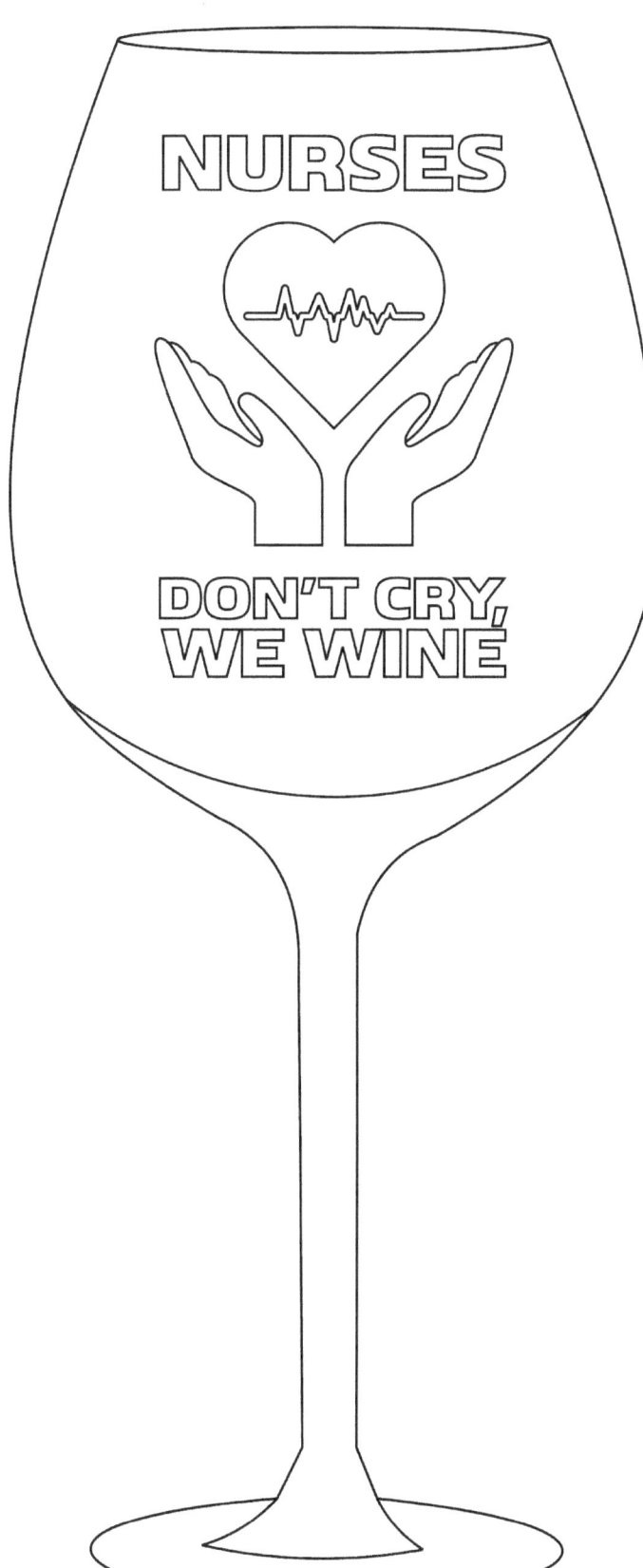

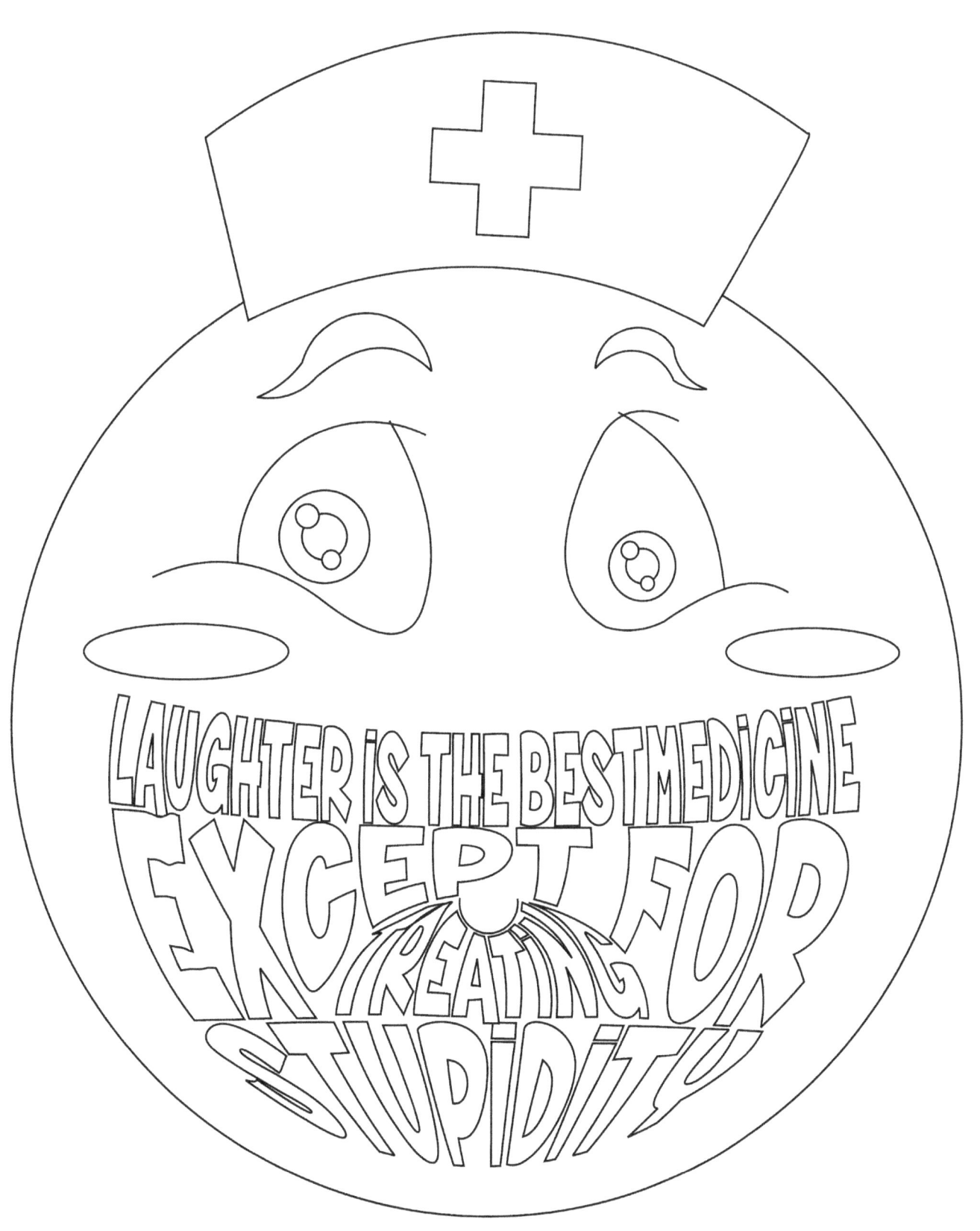

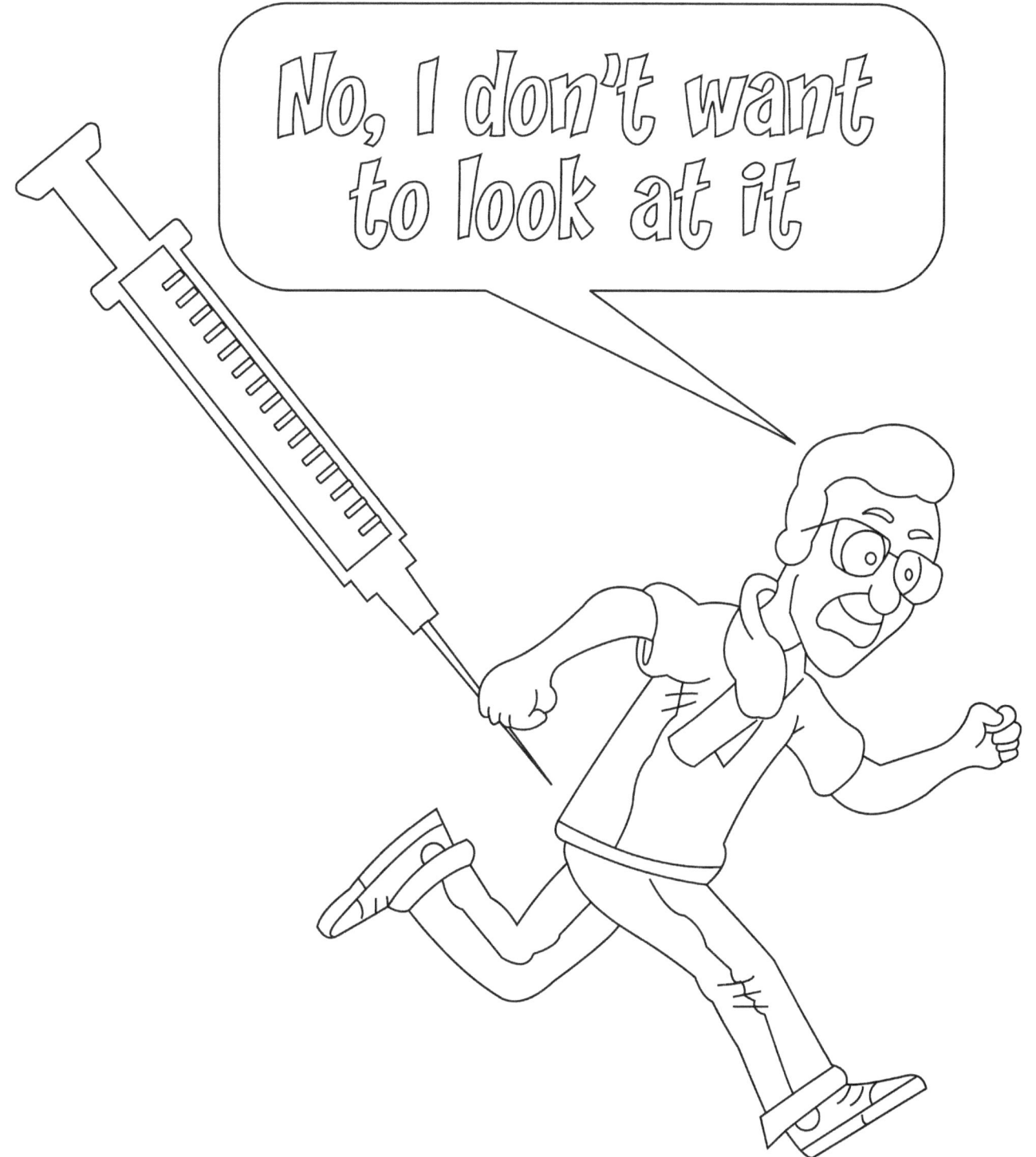

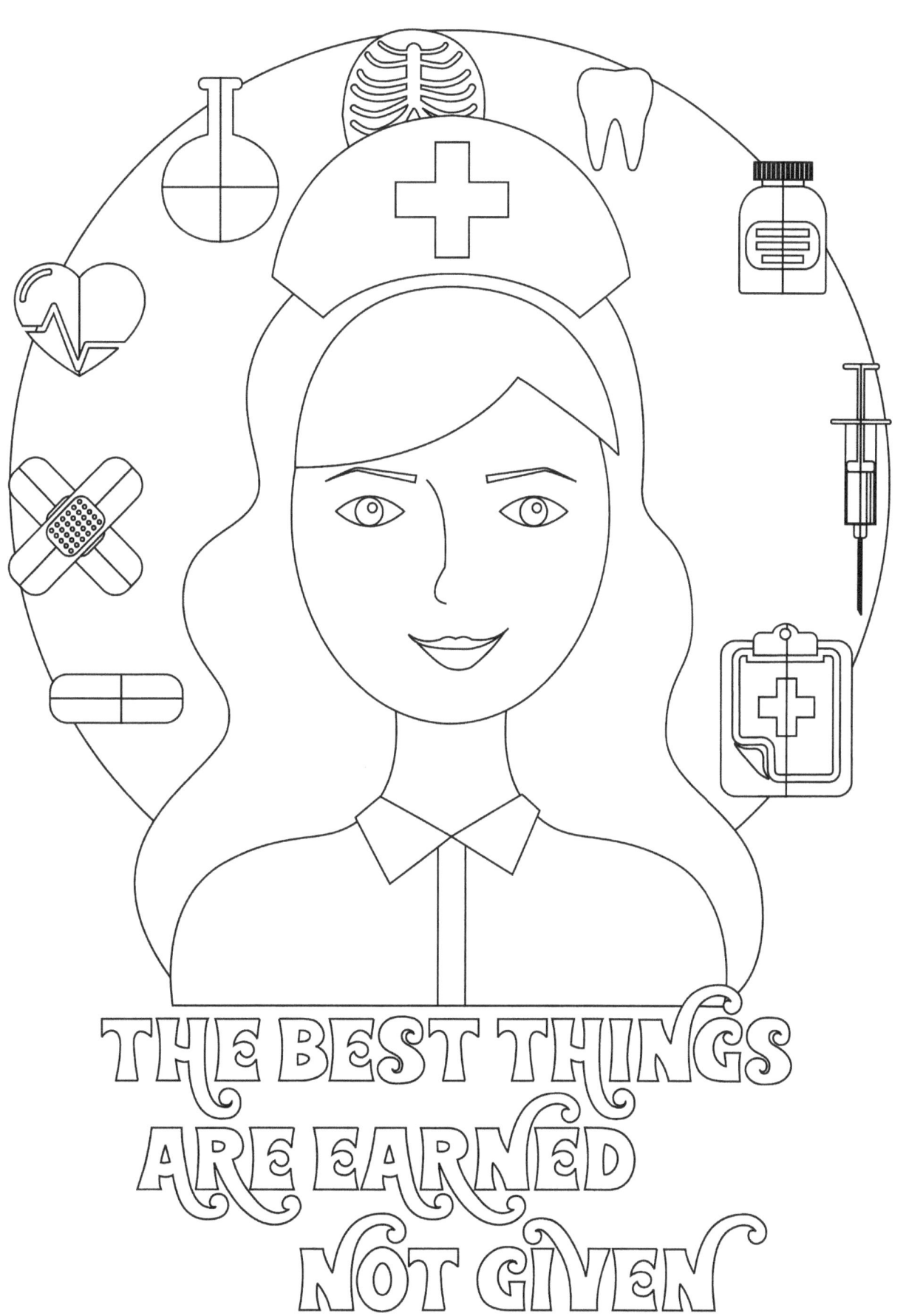

FIXIN' CUTS AND

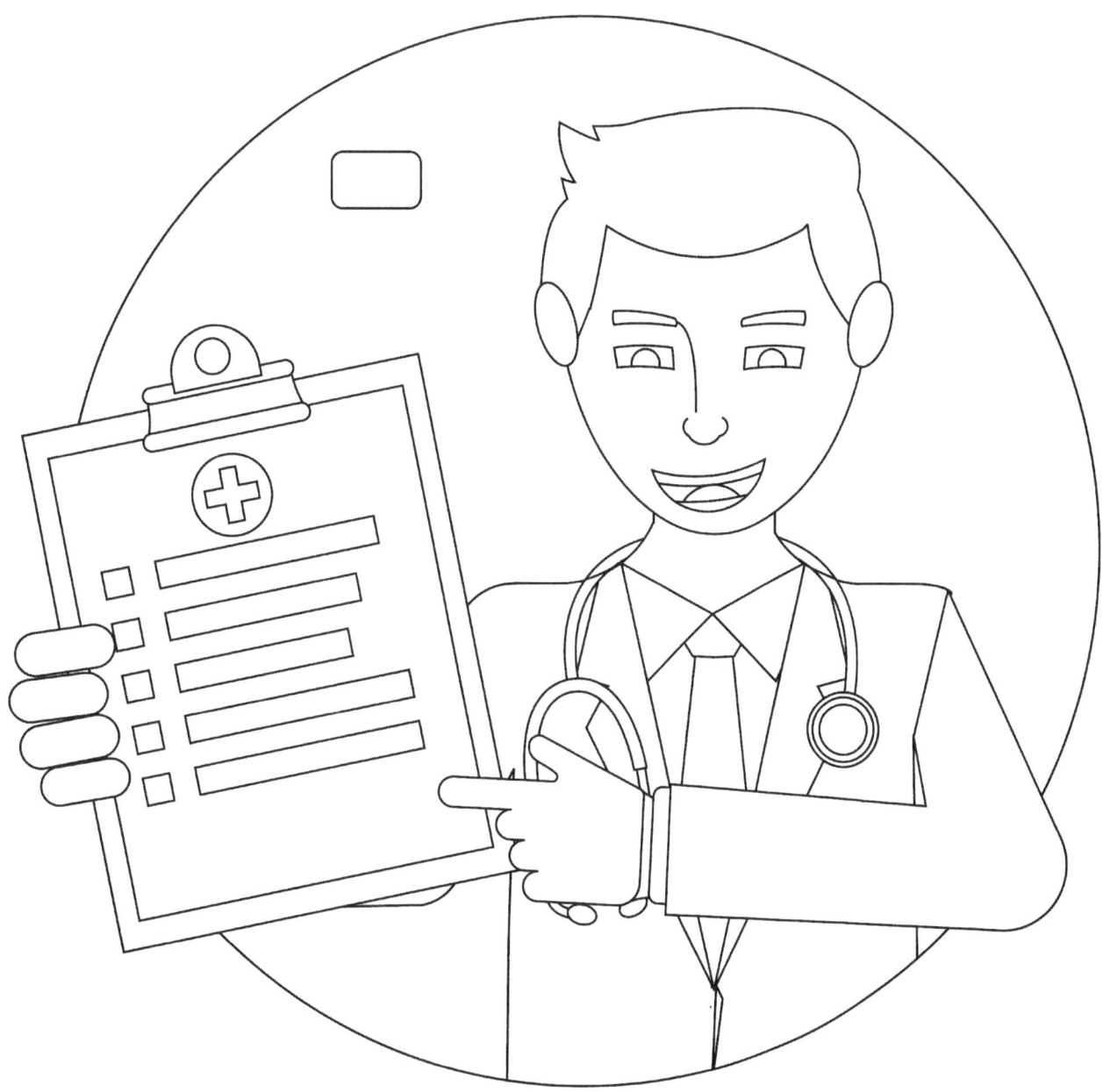

STICKIN' BUTTS

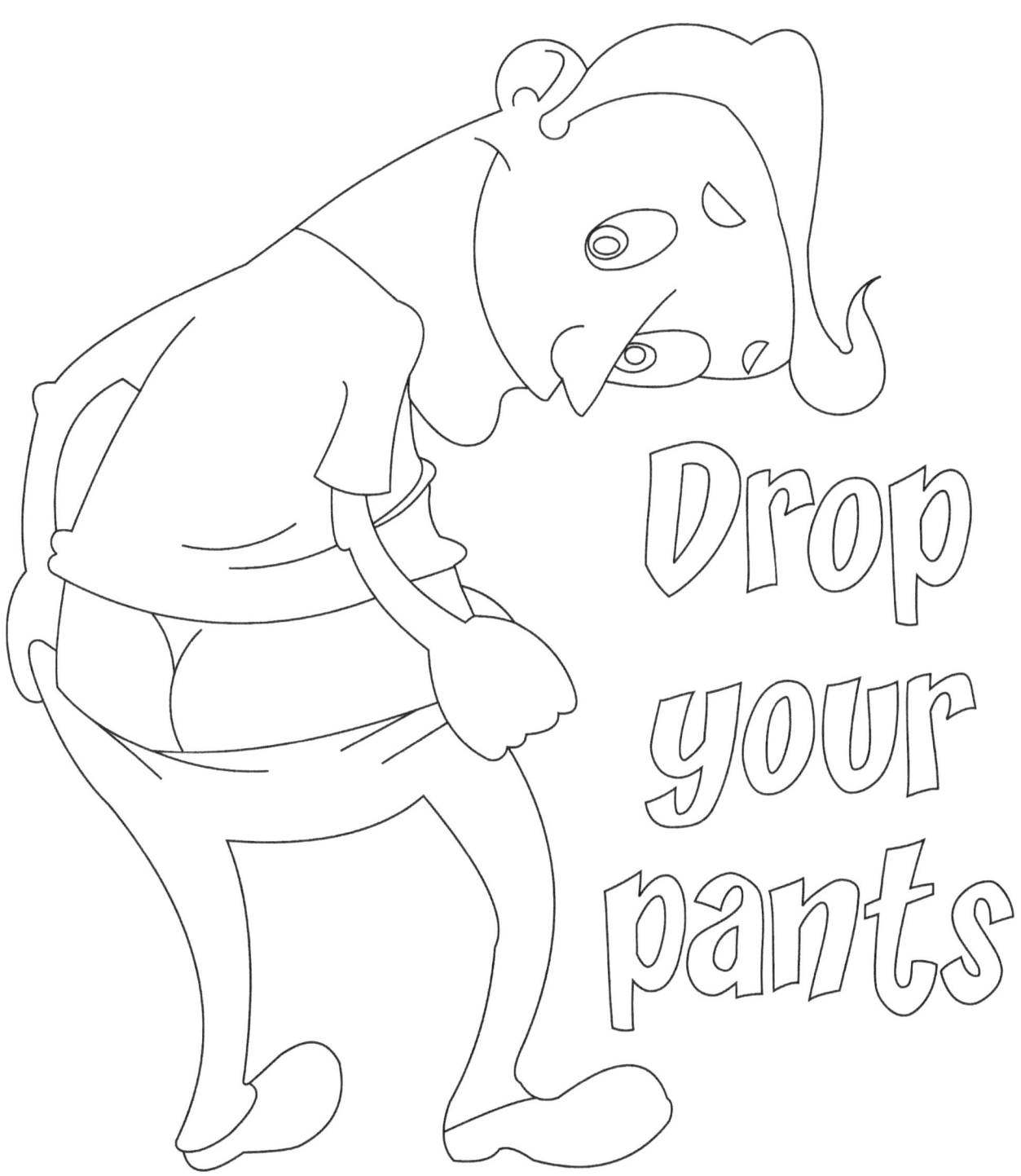

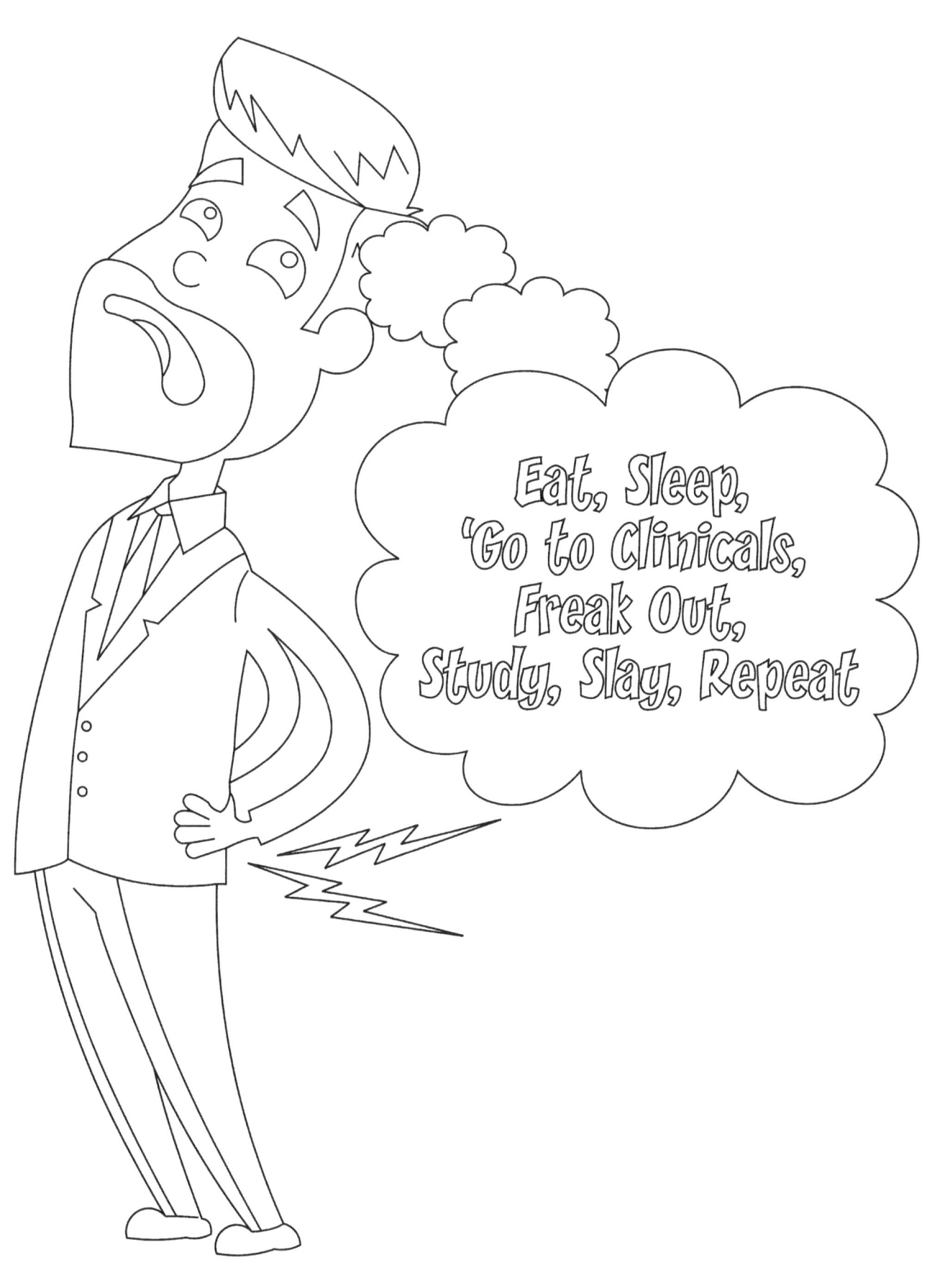

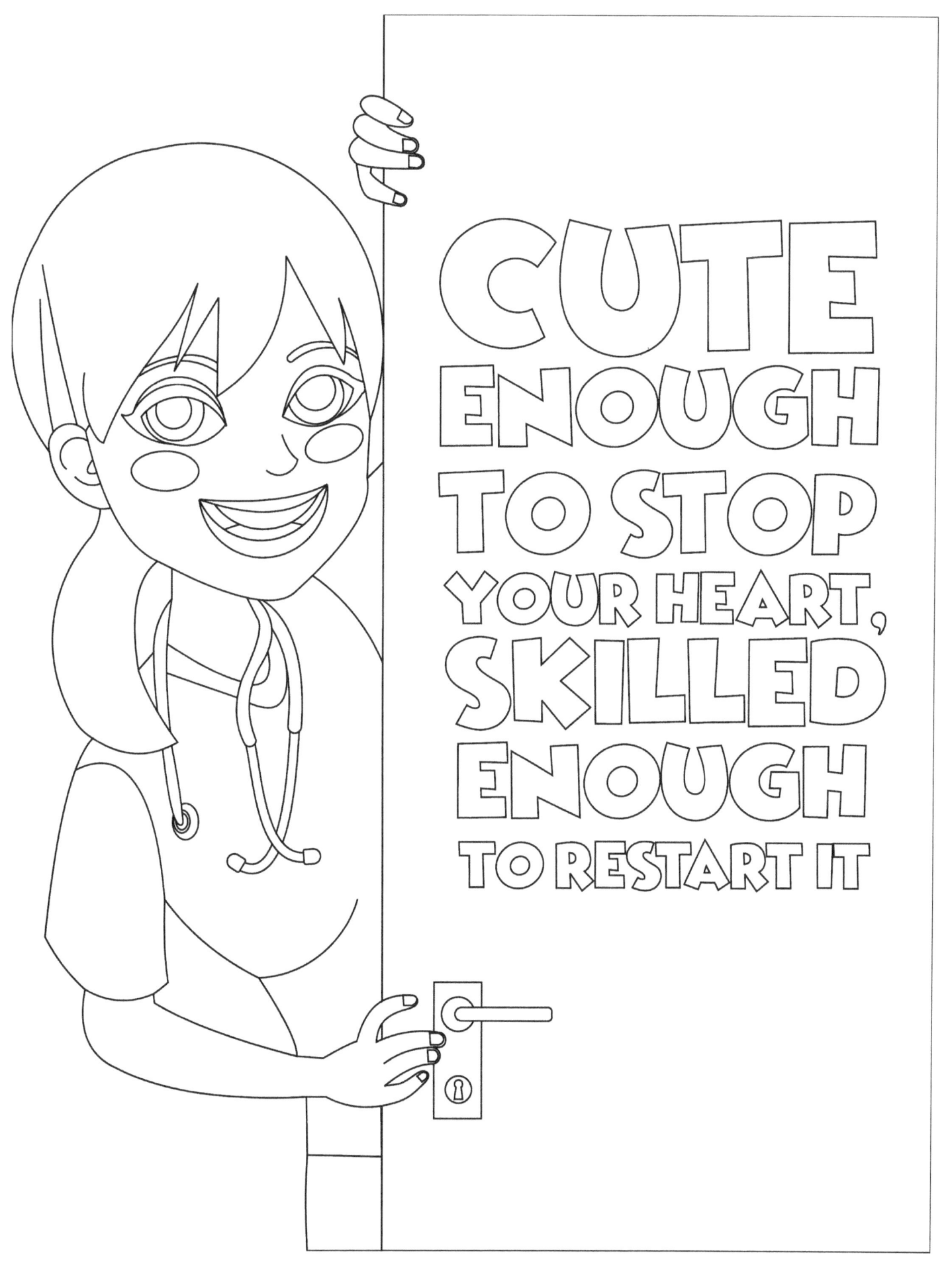

175ml Ethod Po
Tid Prn Stress

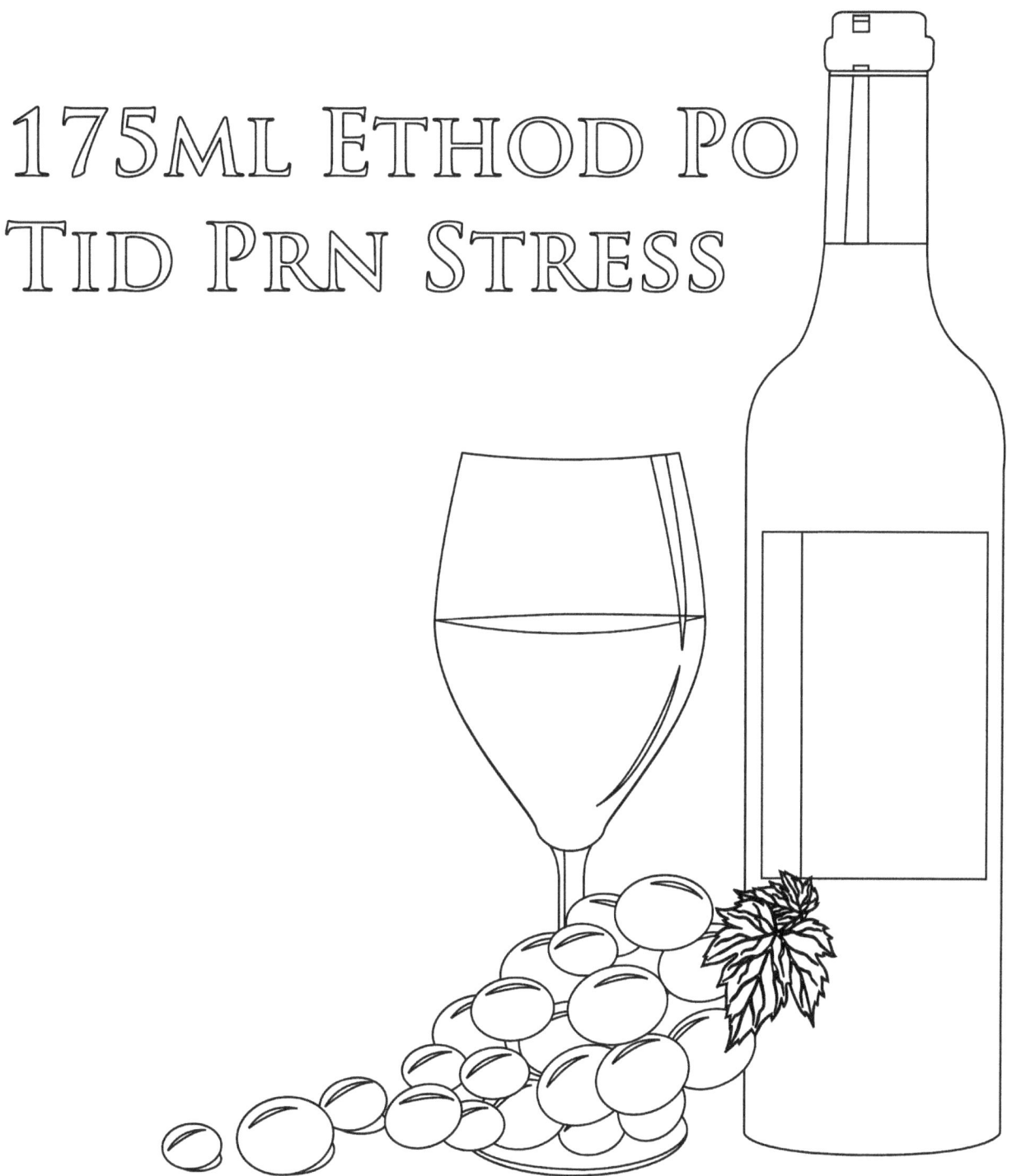

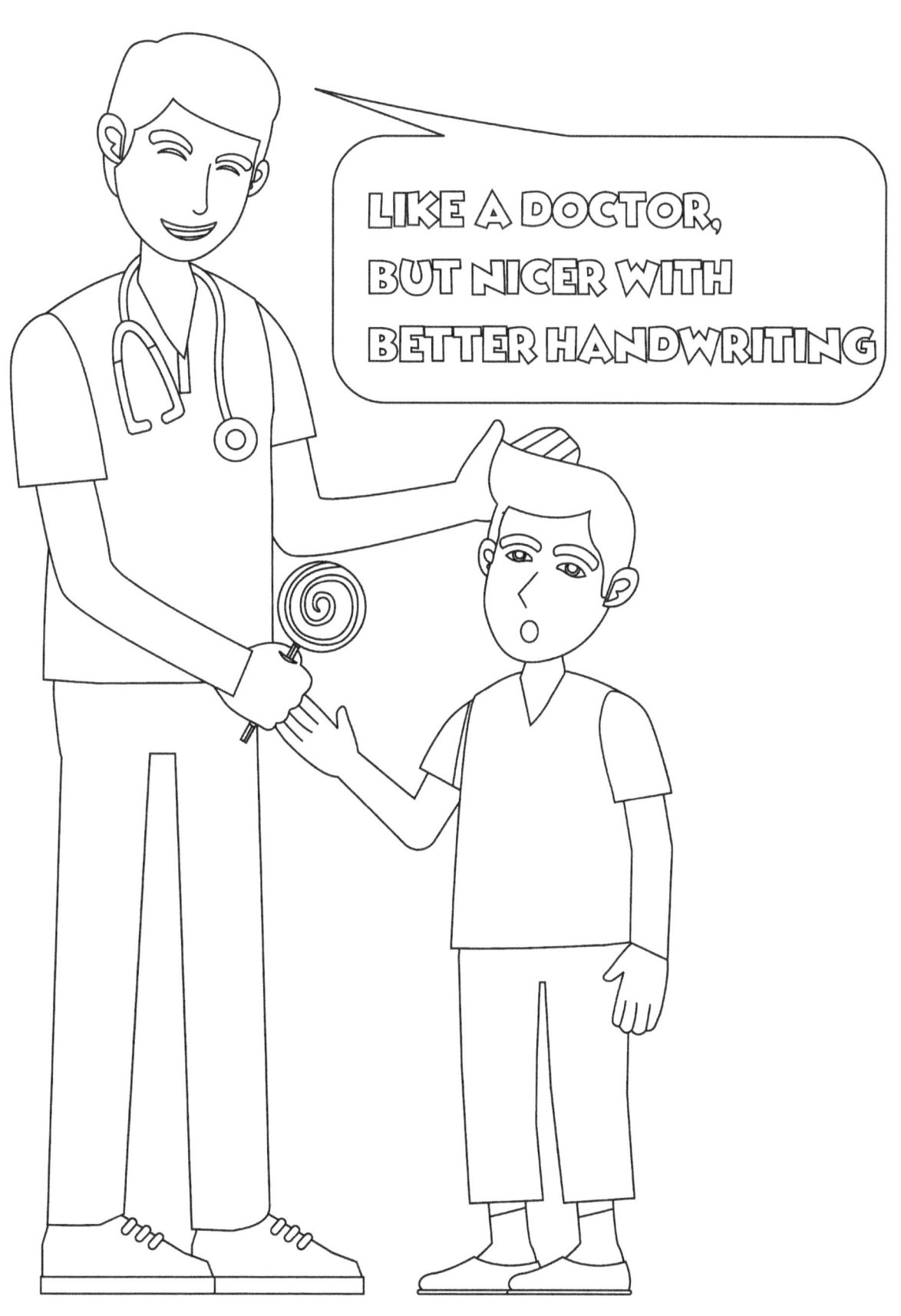

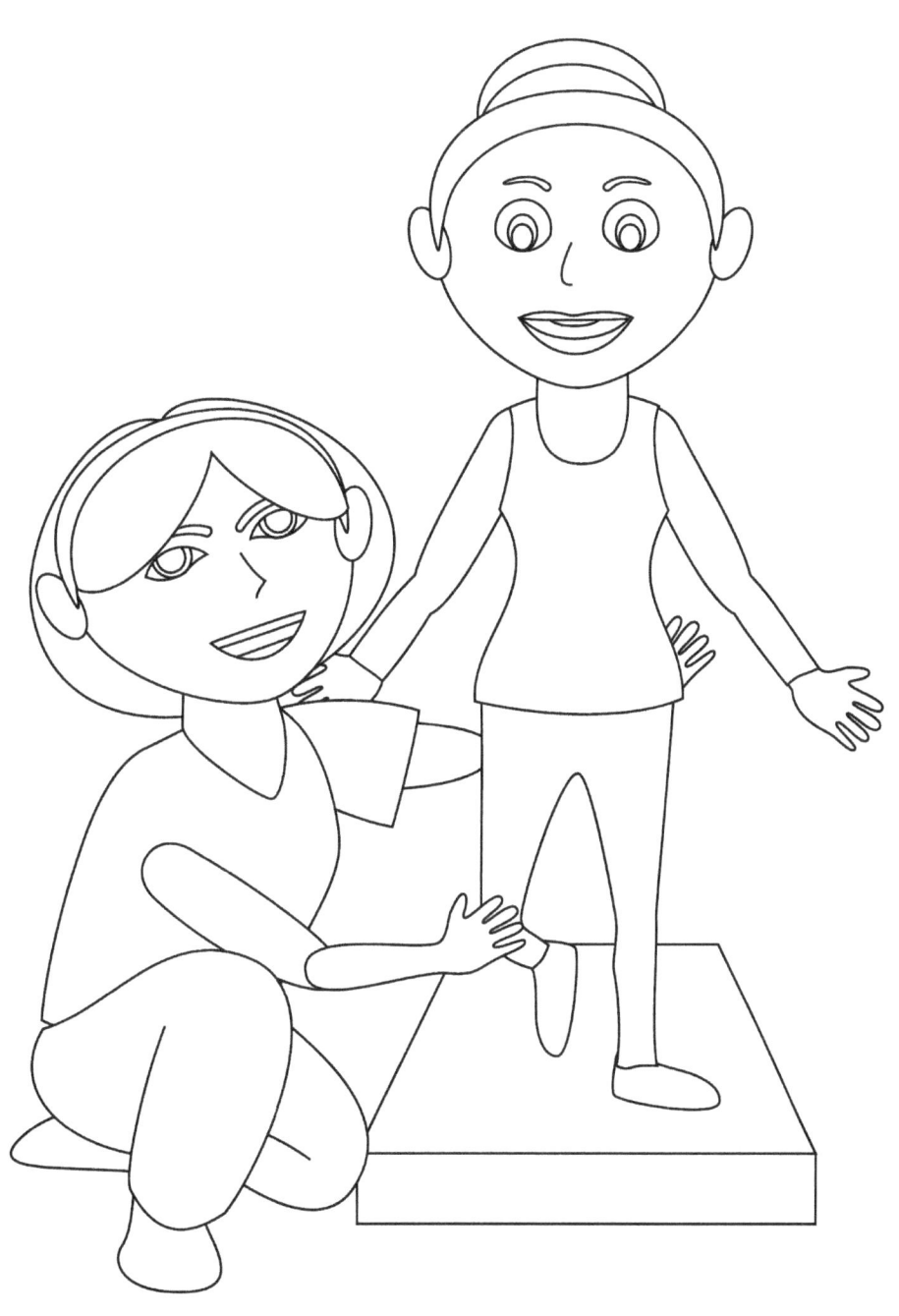

NURSES PATIENT PEOPLE

Nurse
survival 101:

Caffenie
before shift

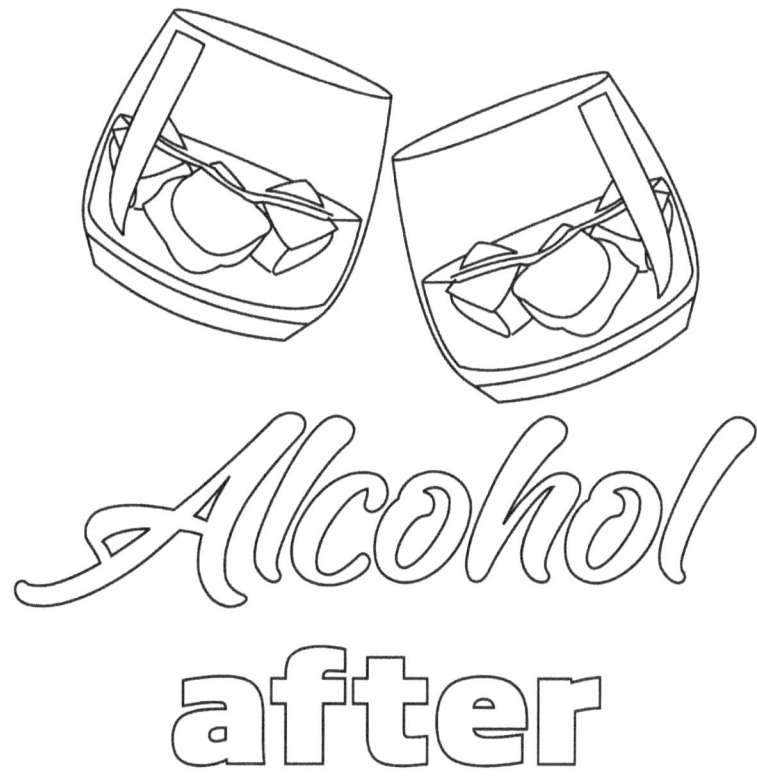

Alcohol
after

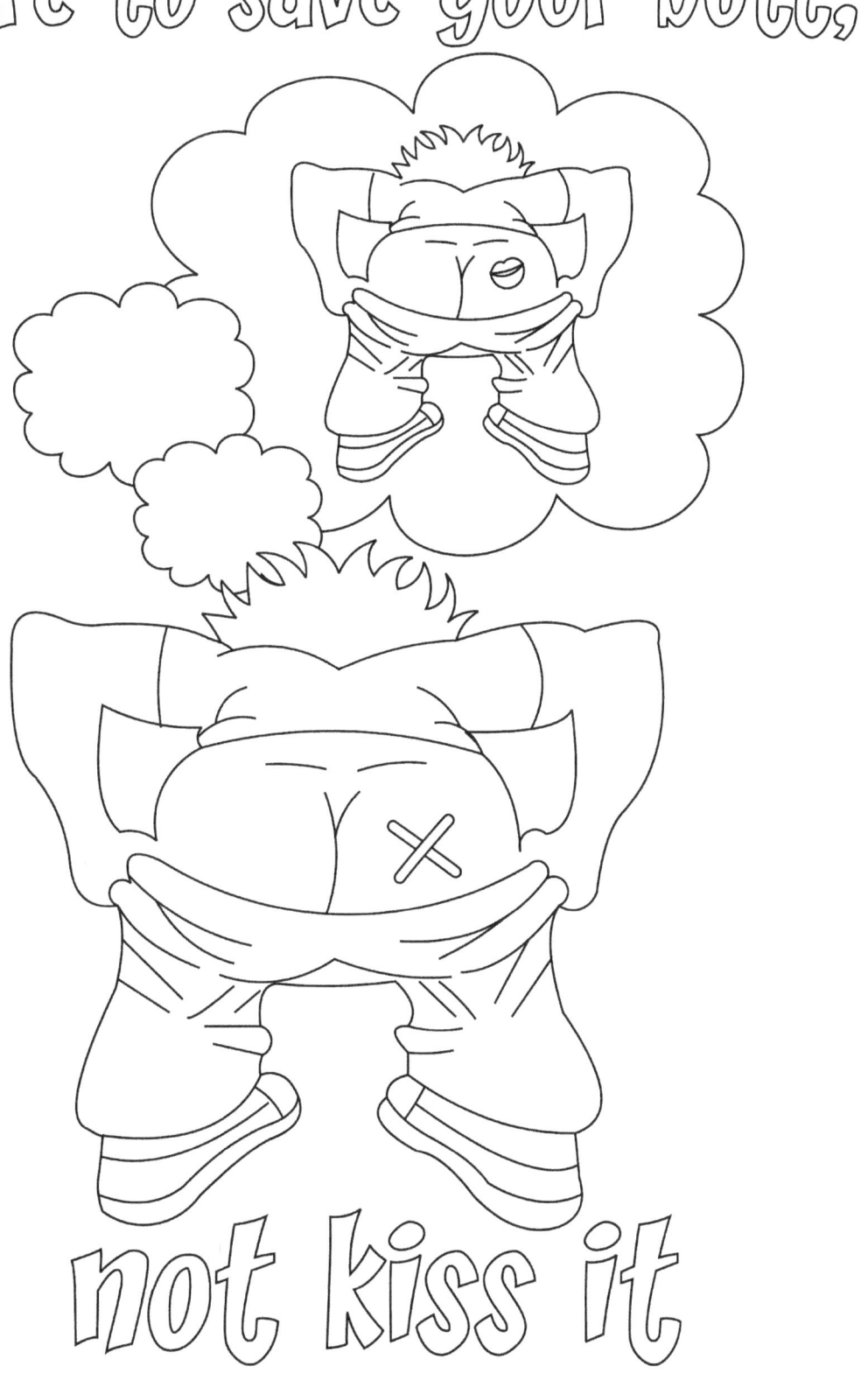

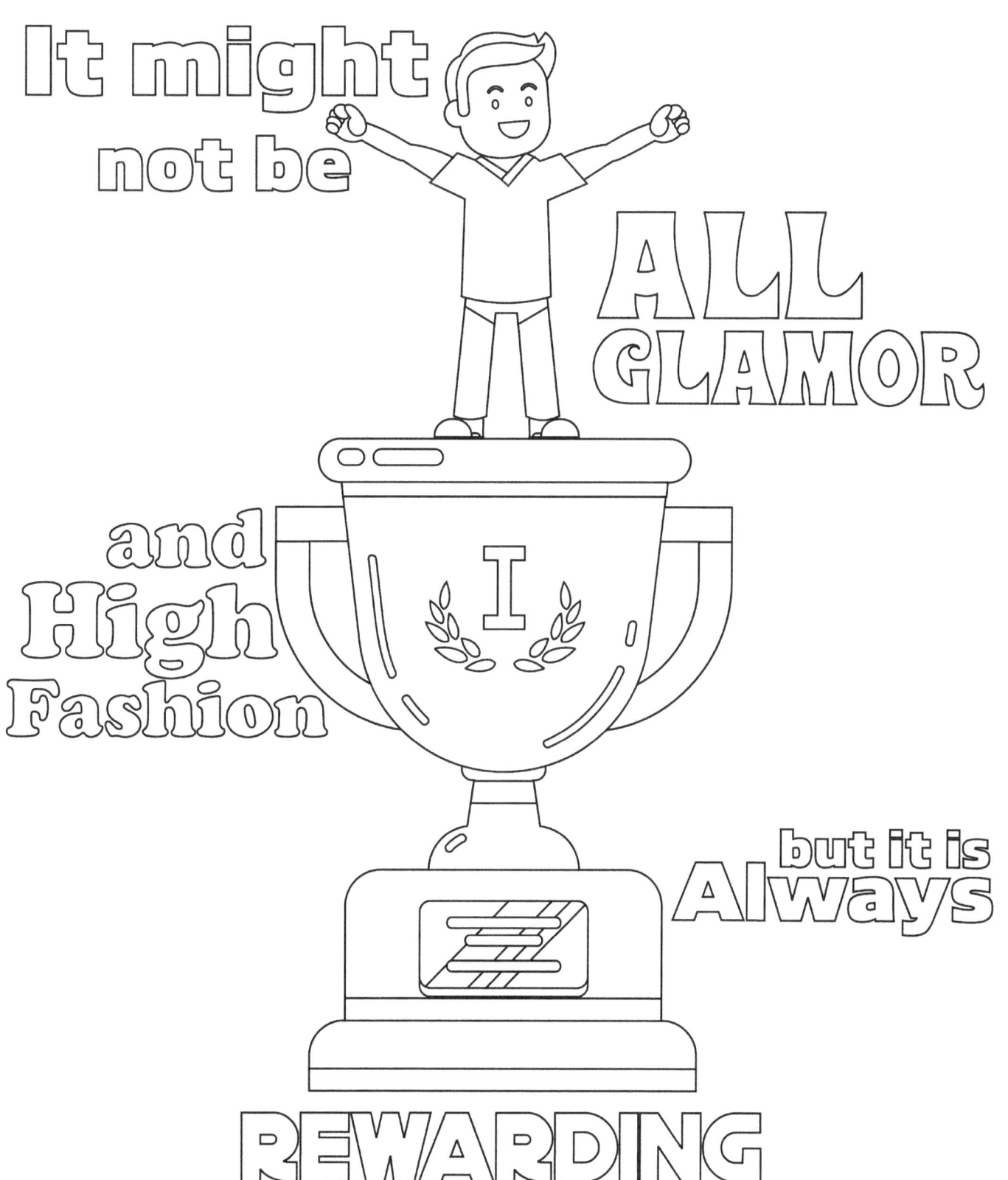

A patient almost died in front of me, but then I counted 10 and put the scissors back in my pocket

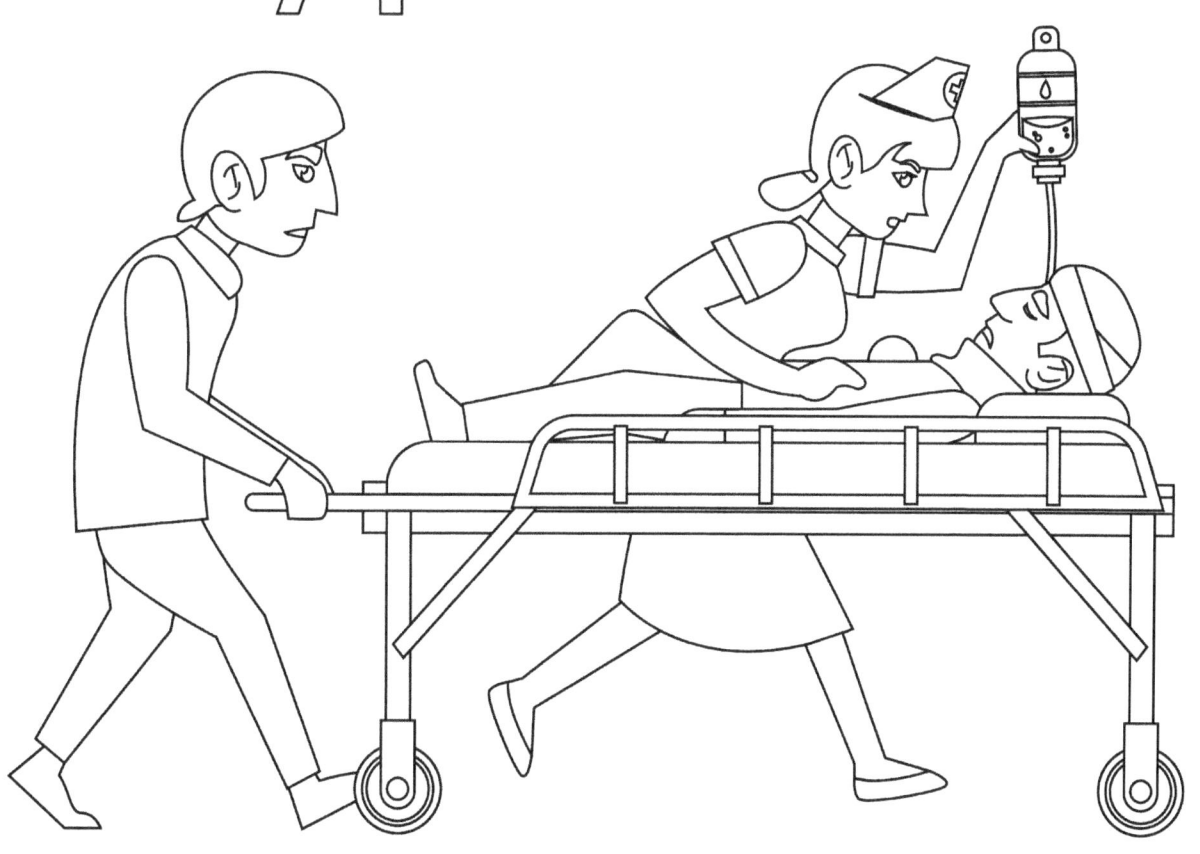

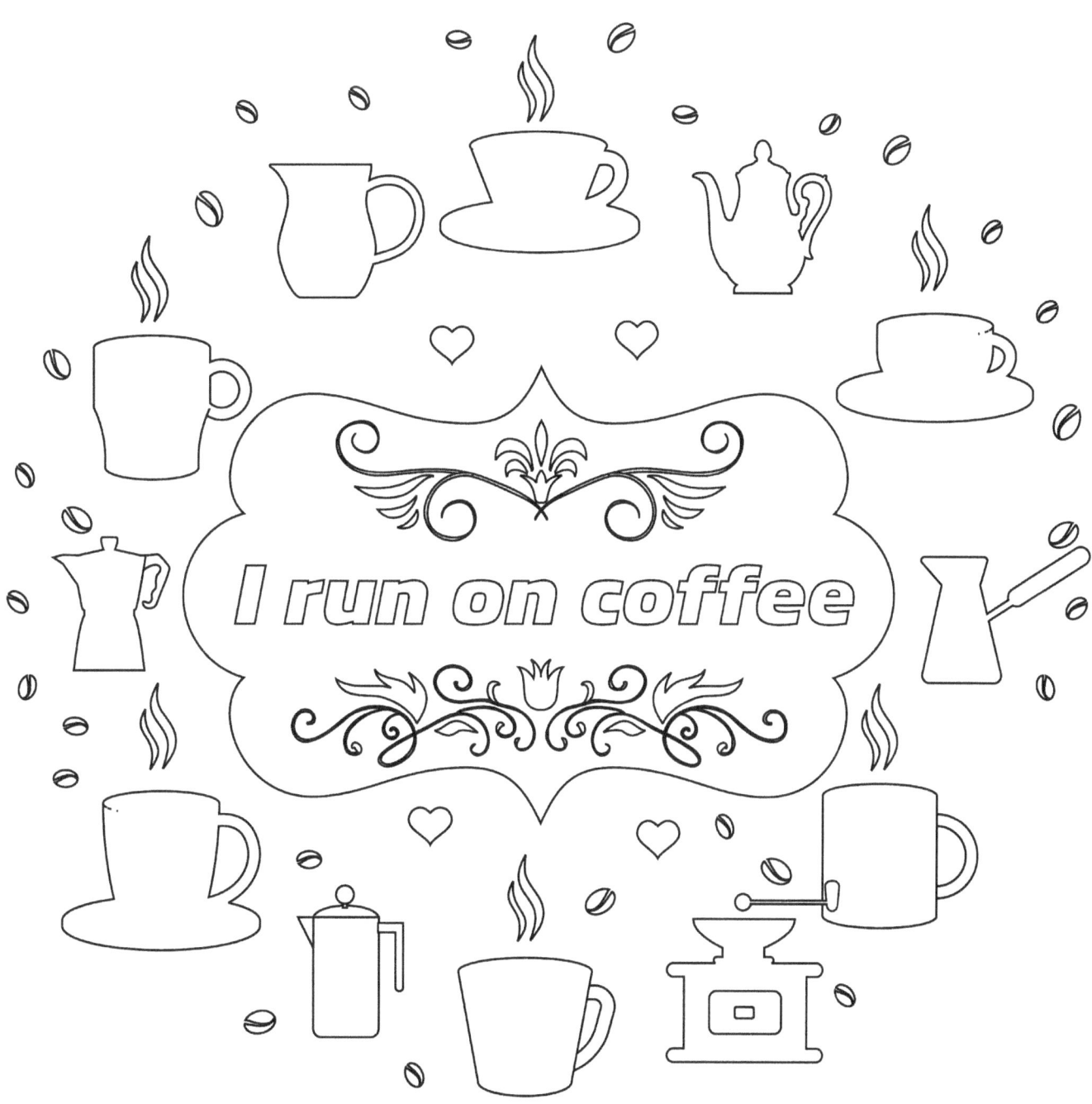

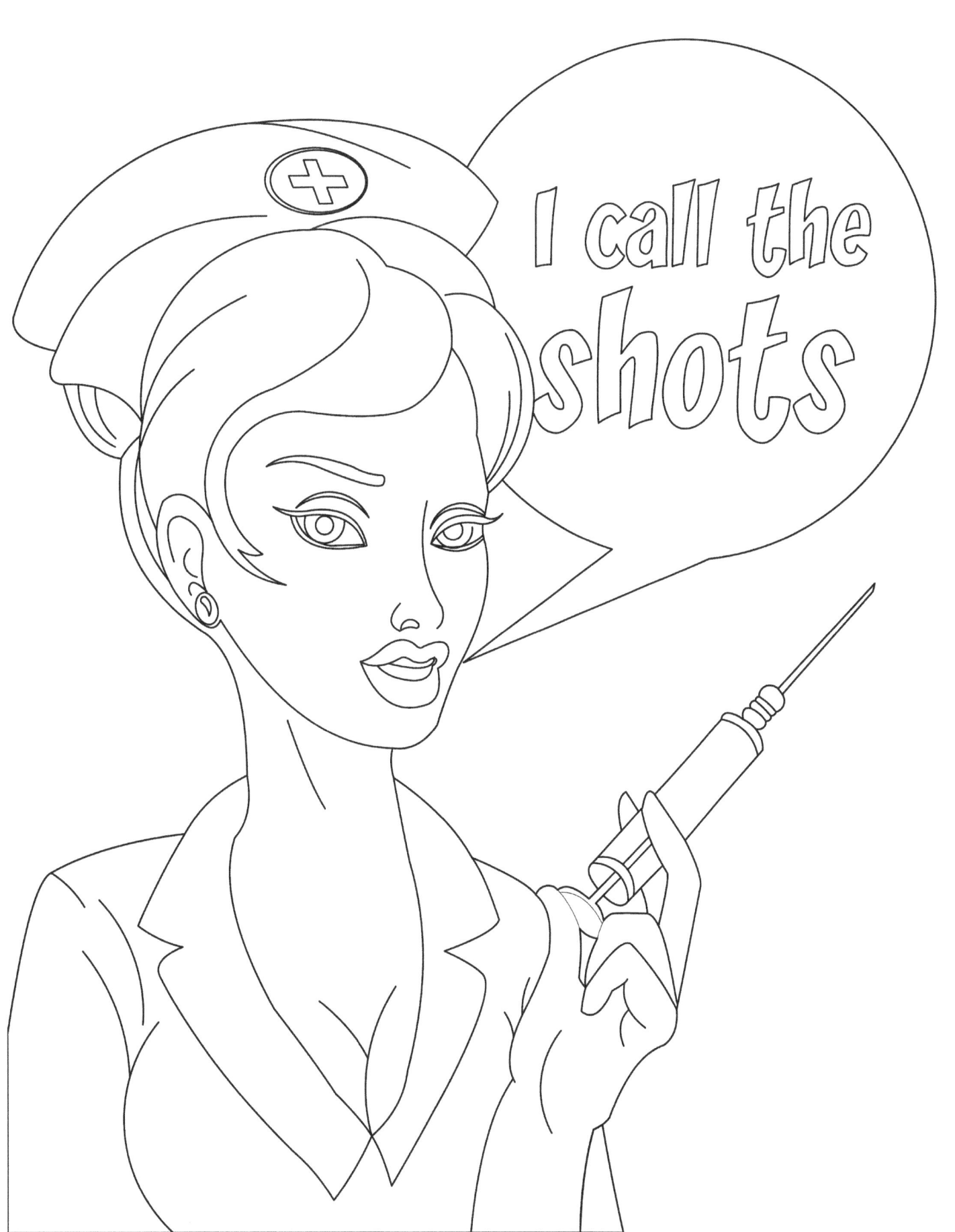

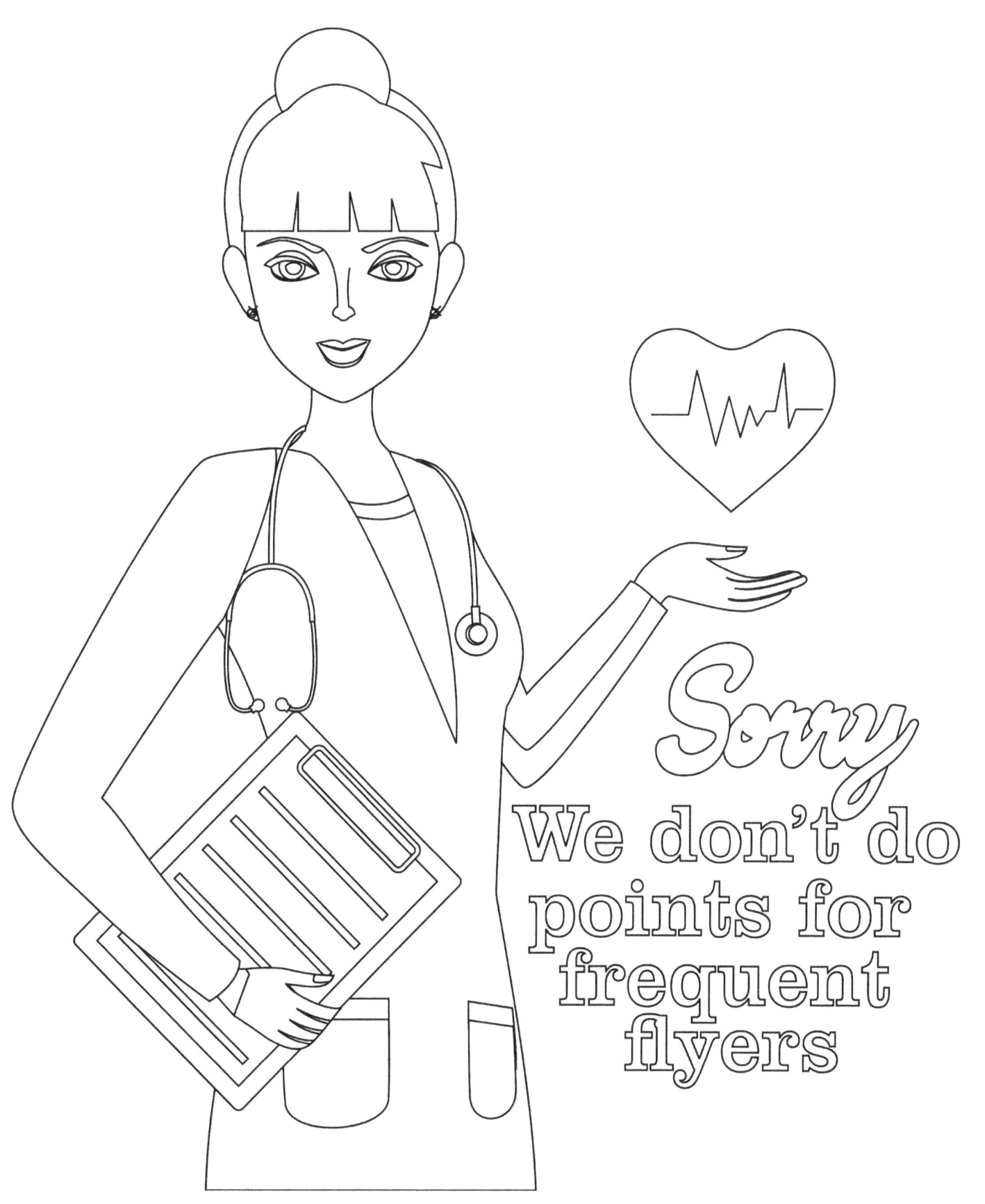

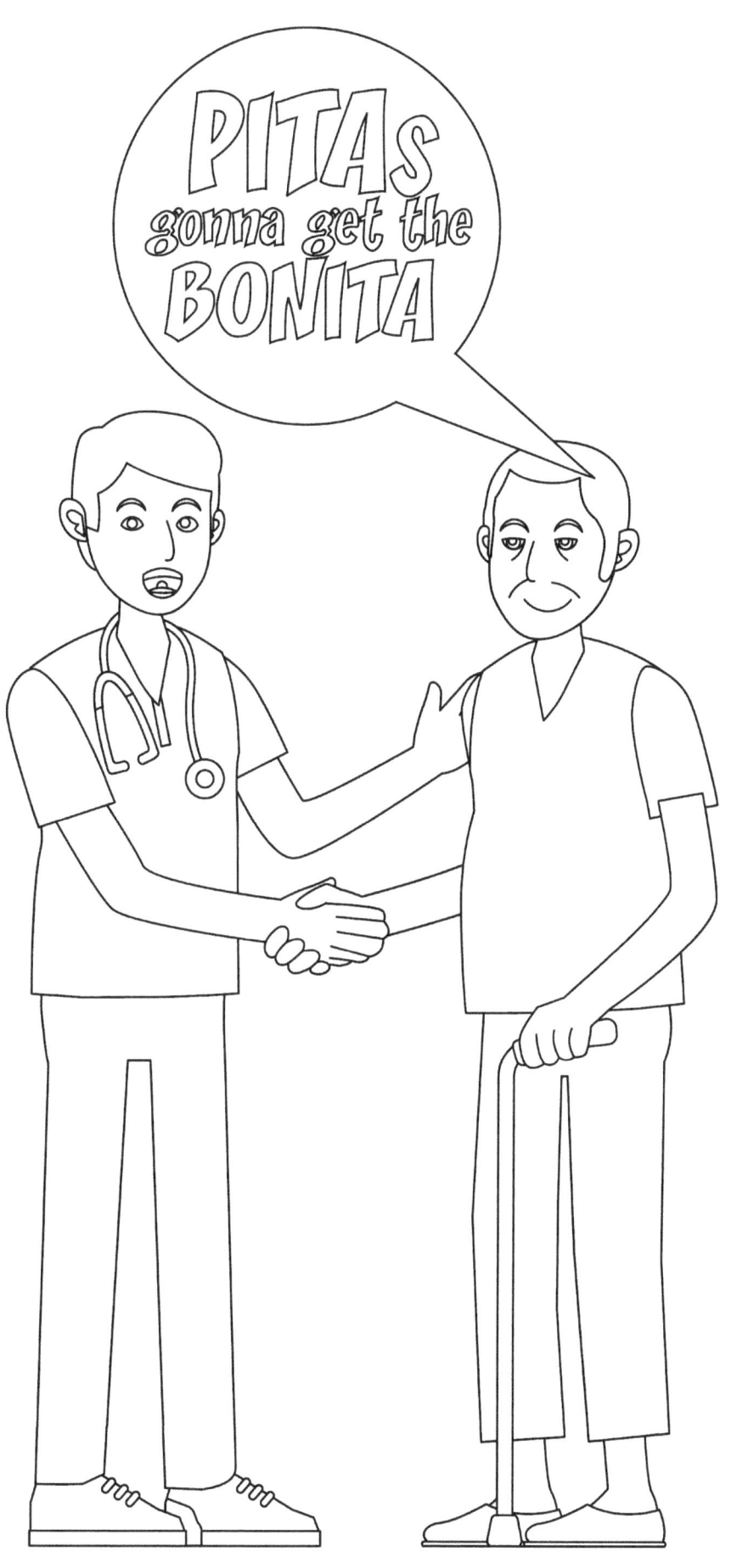

Remember,
I choose the size of the catheters and needles!

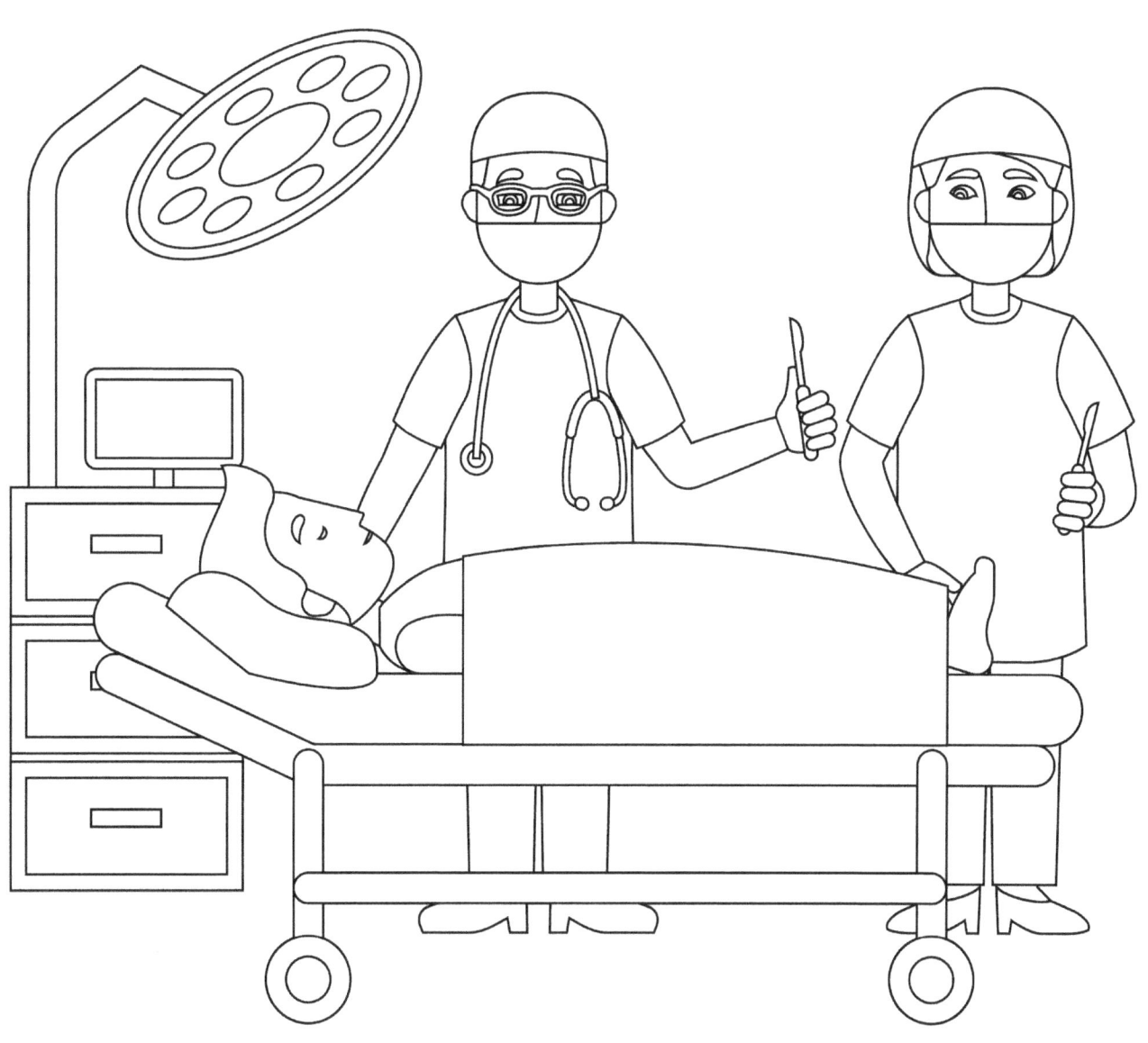

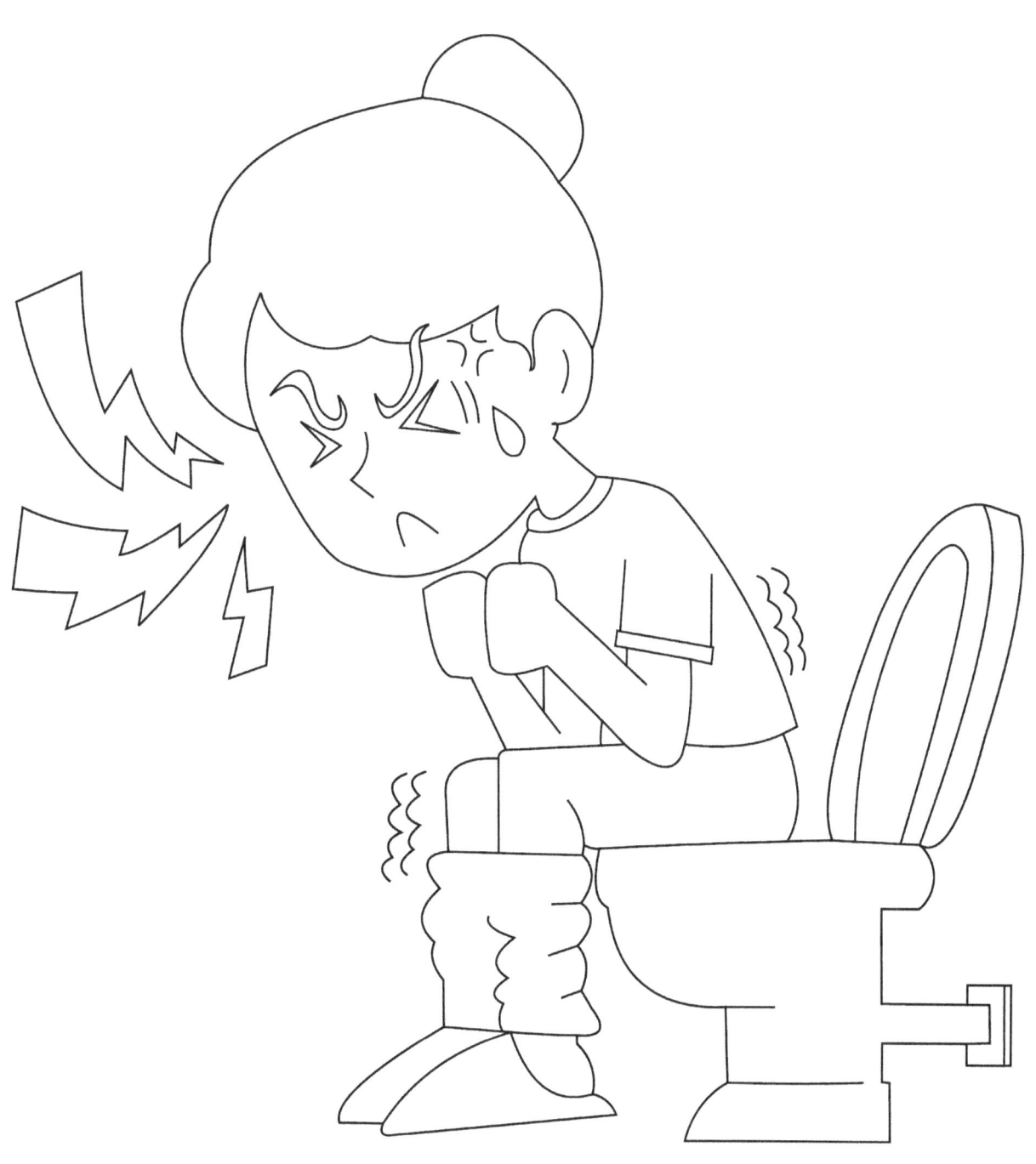

Dear status dramaticus, the crying with no tears and complaints of 10/10 pain are only fooling your enabling family

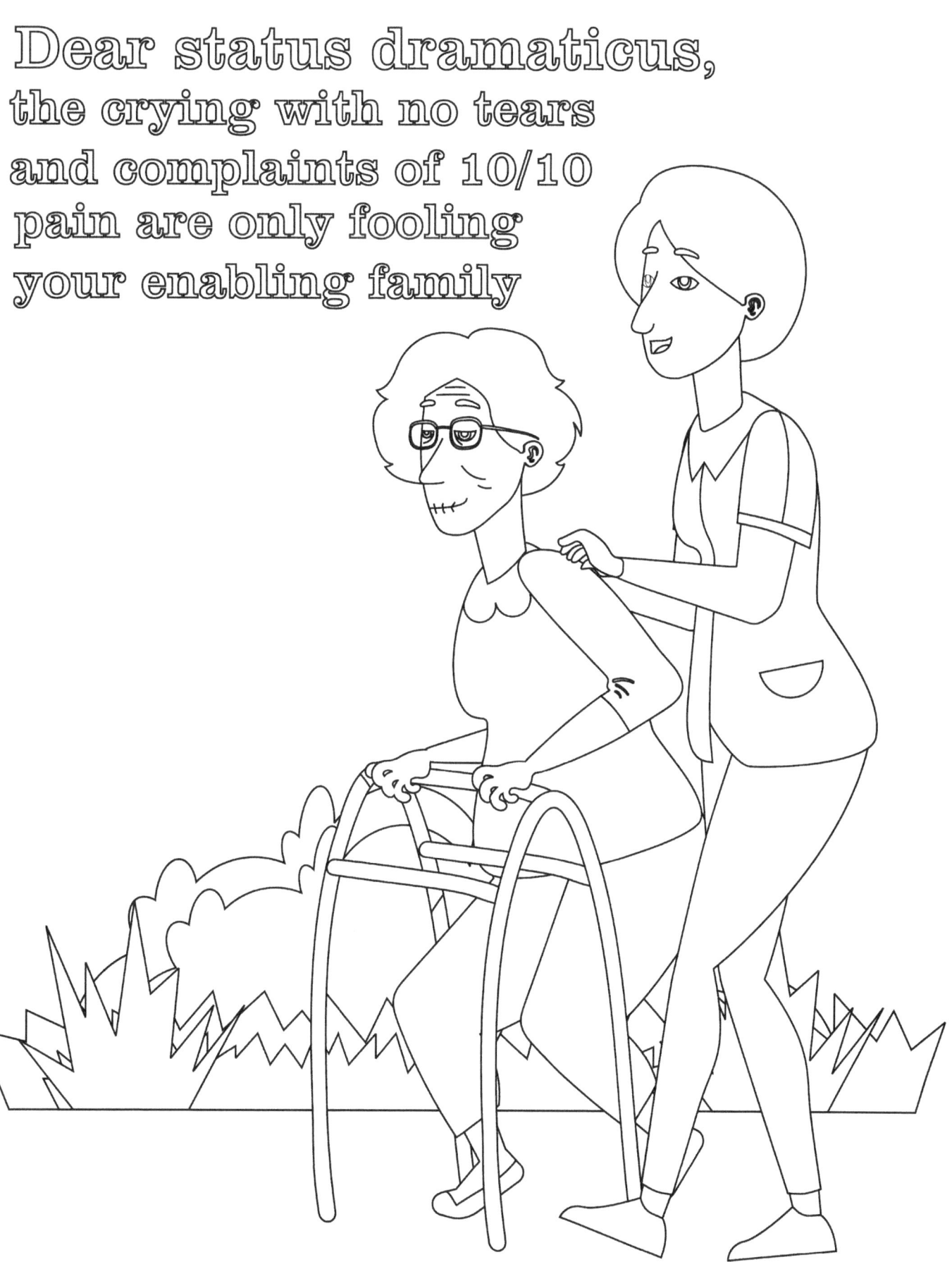

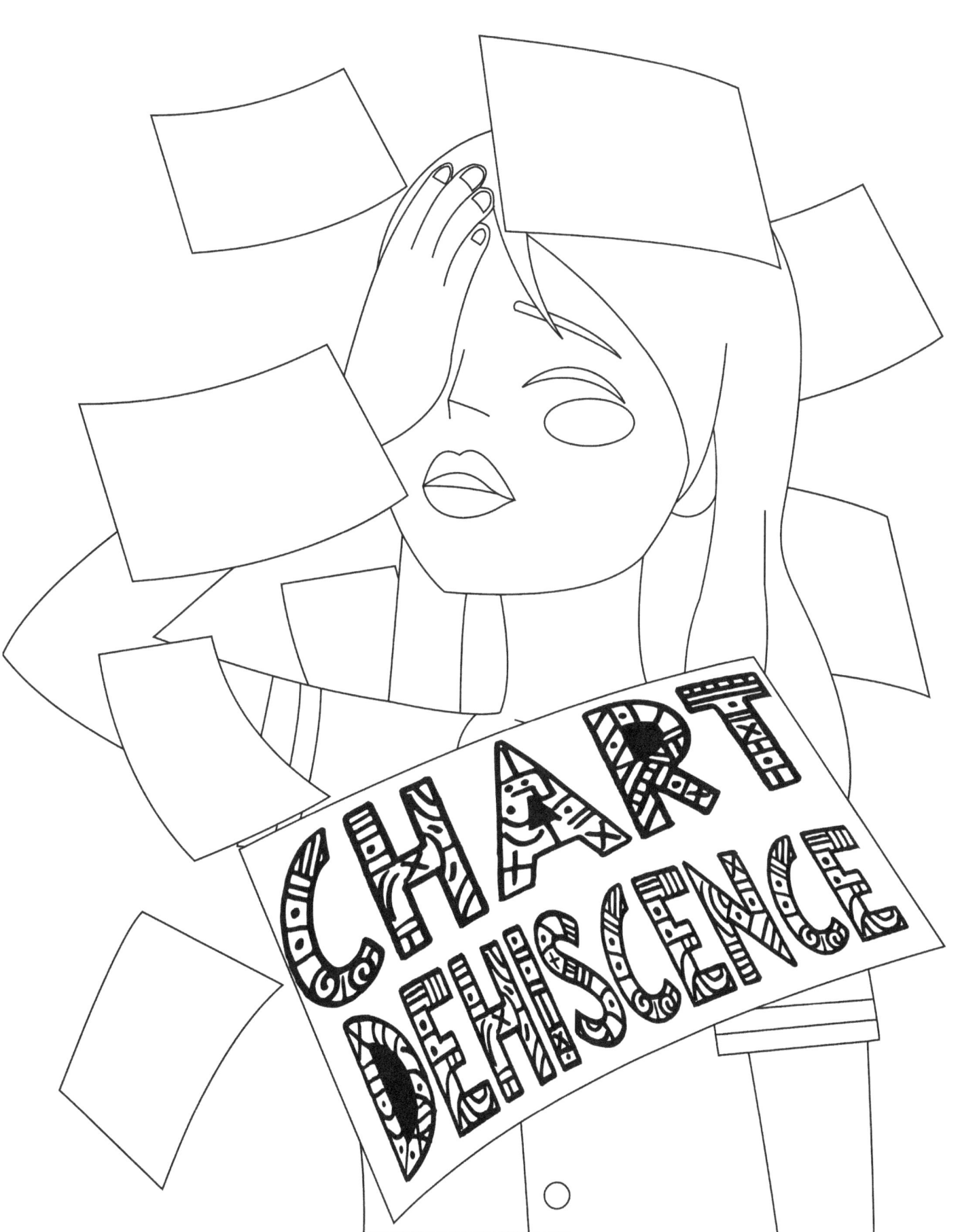

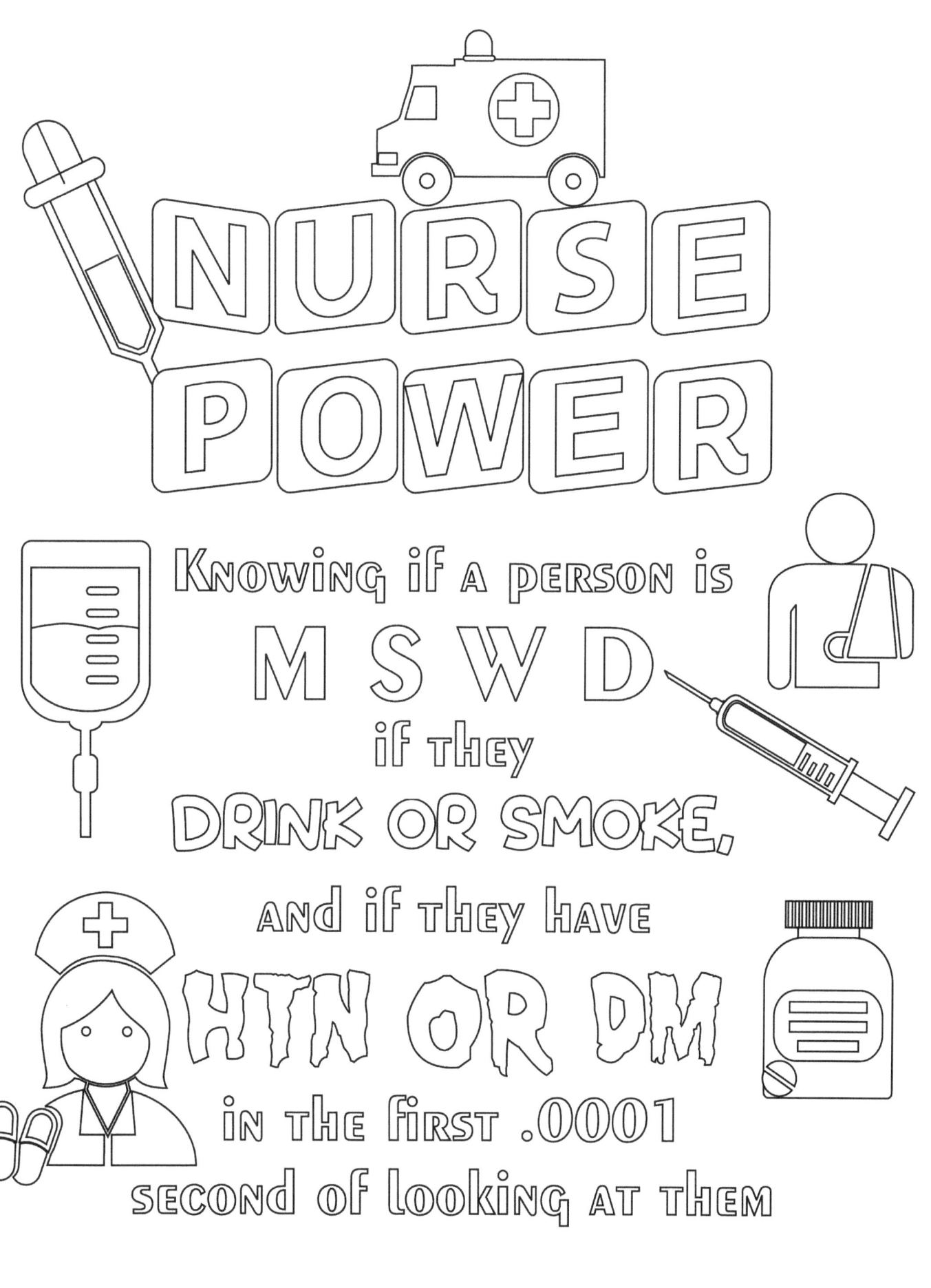

NURSE LIES:
THIS WON'T HURT A BIT

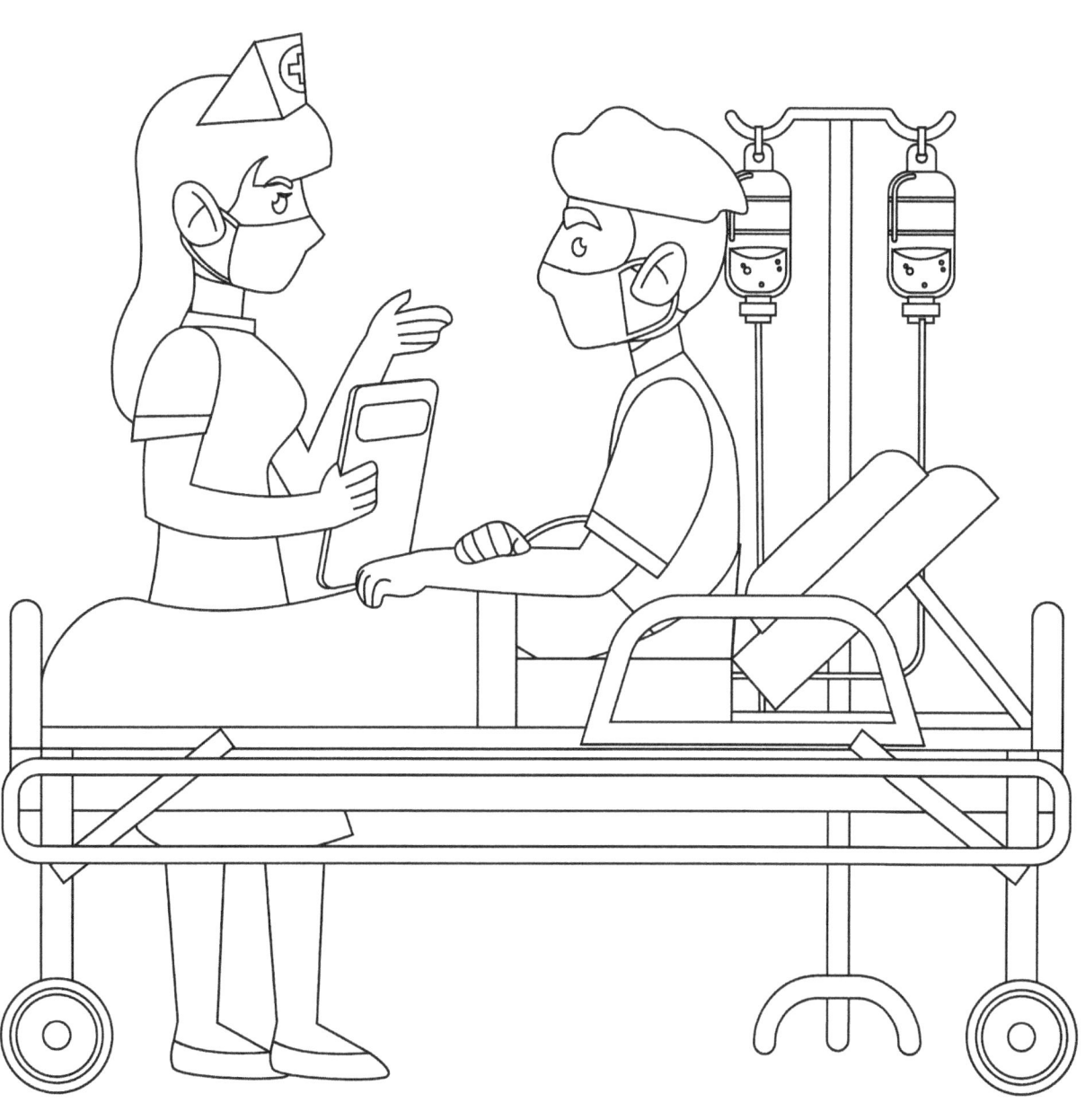

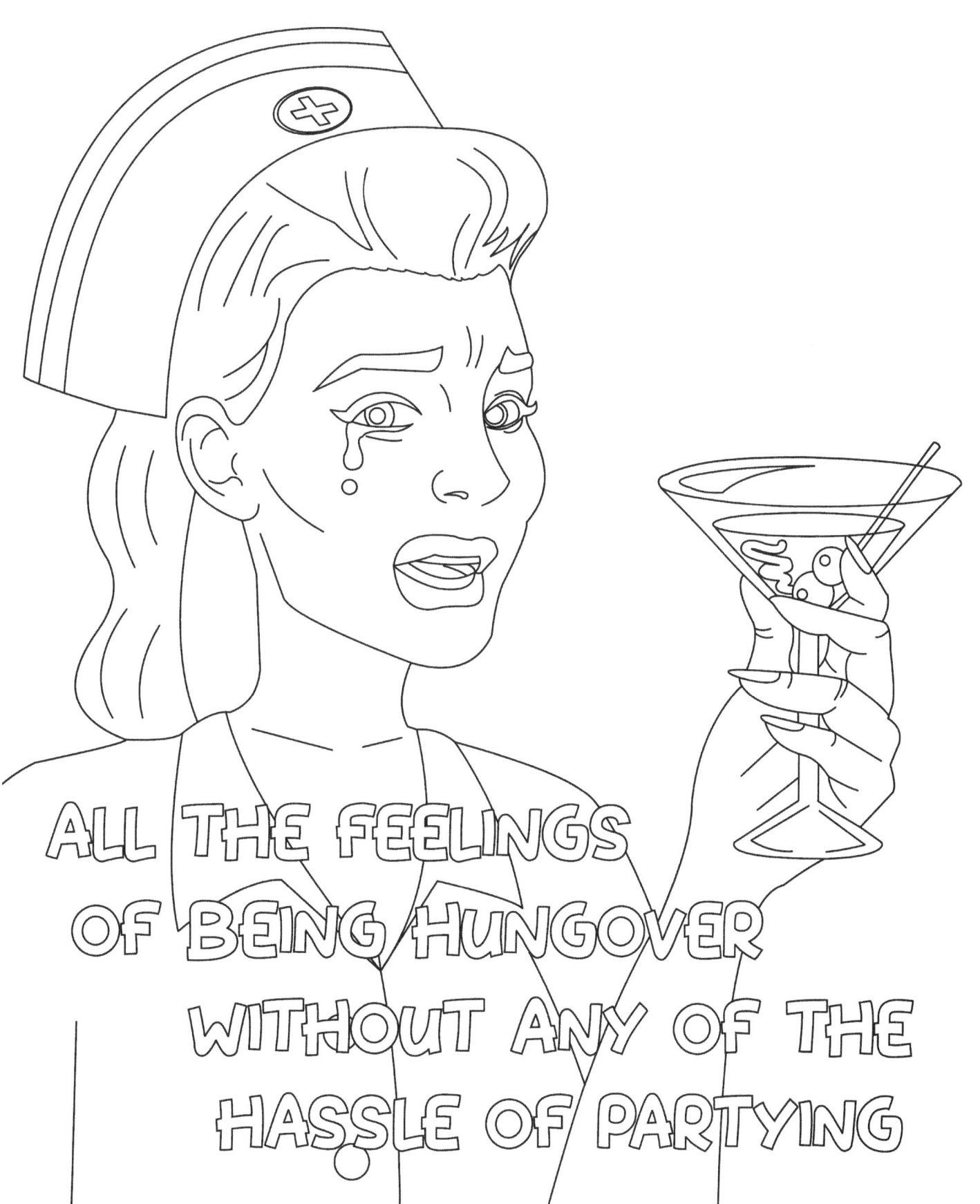

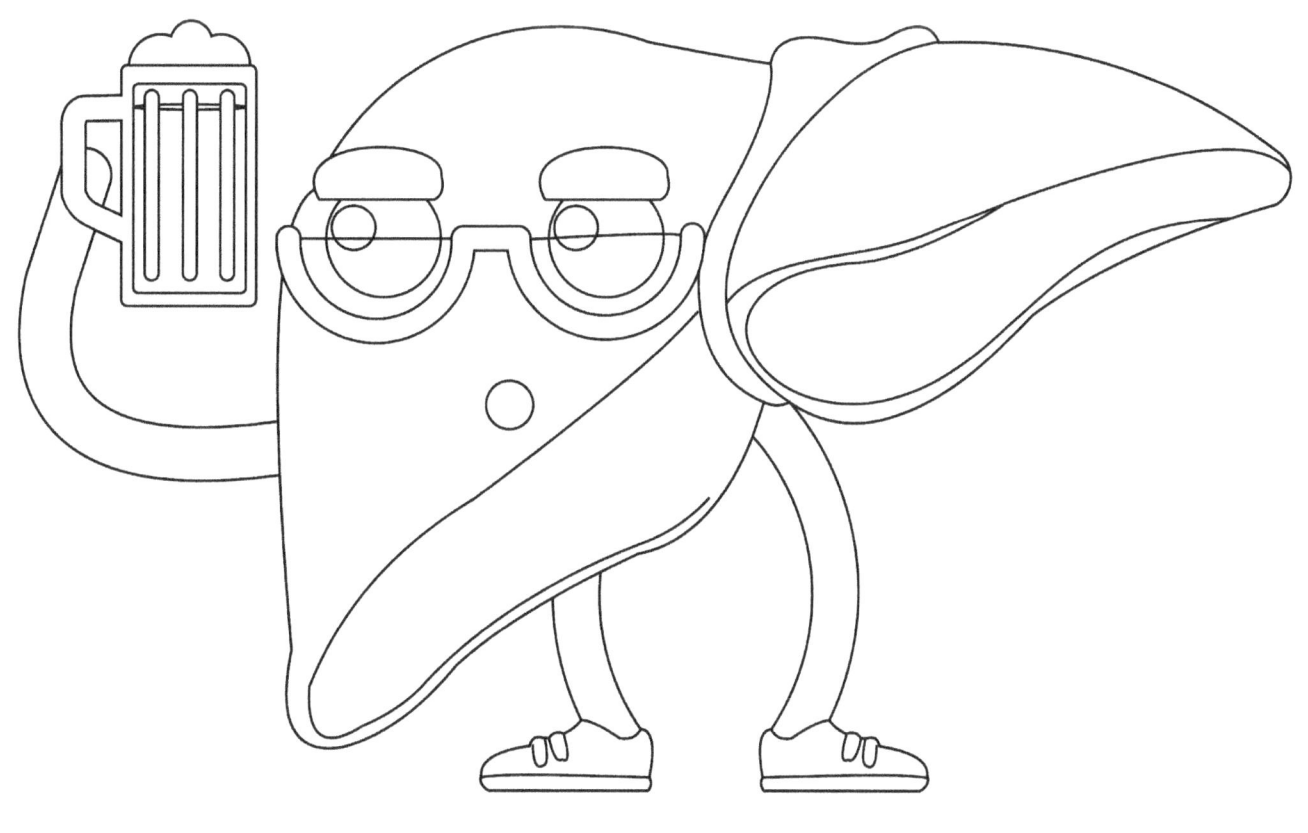

You say alcoholism,
I say liver crossfit

I'VE SEEN MORE BUSH THAN A LANDSCAPER HAS

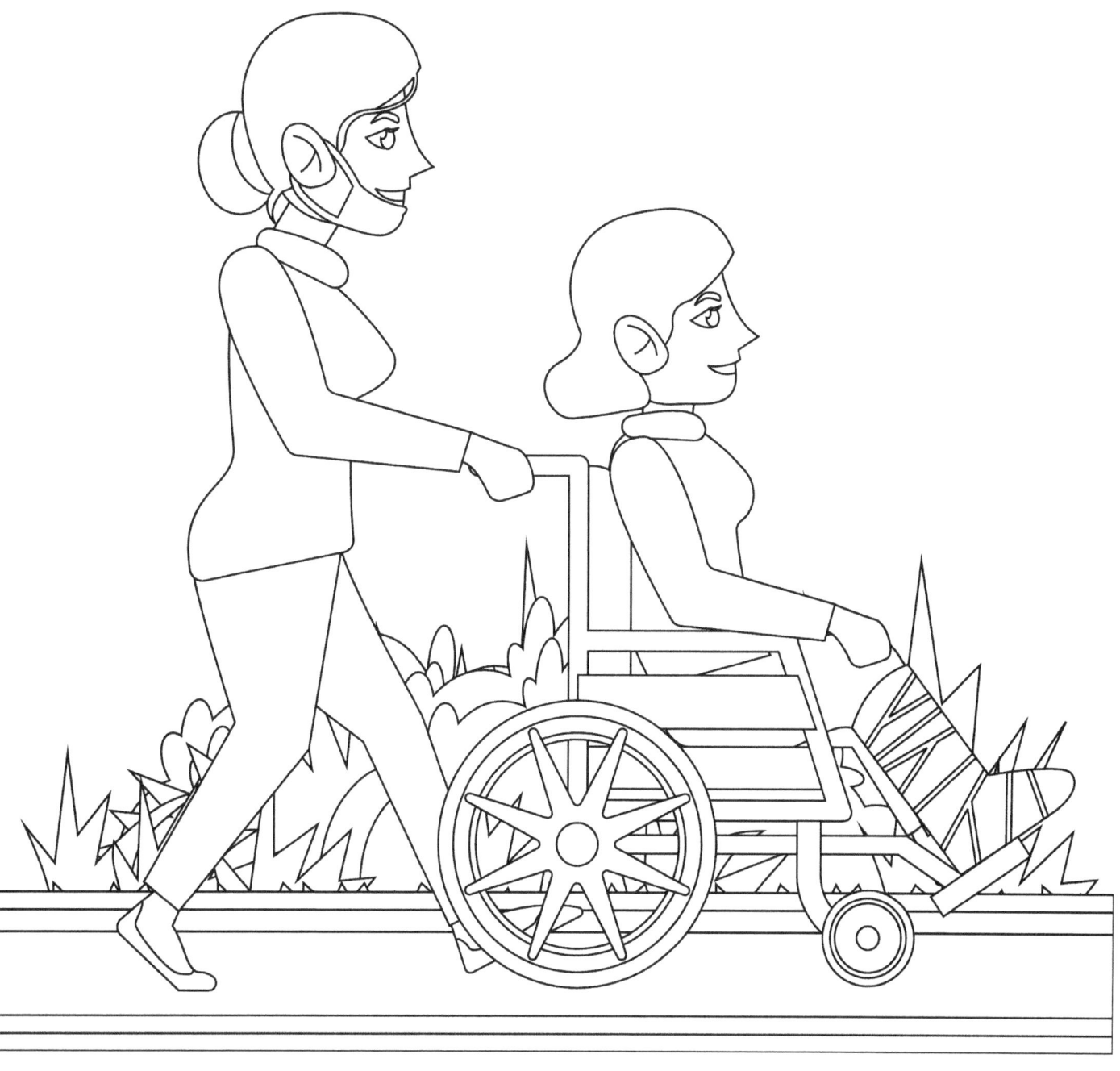

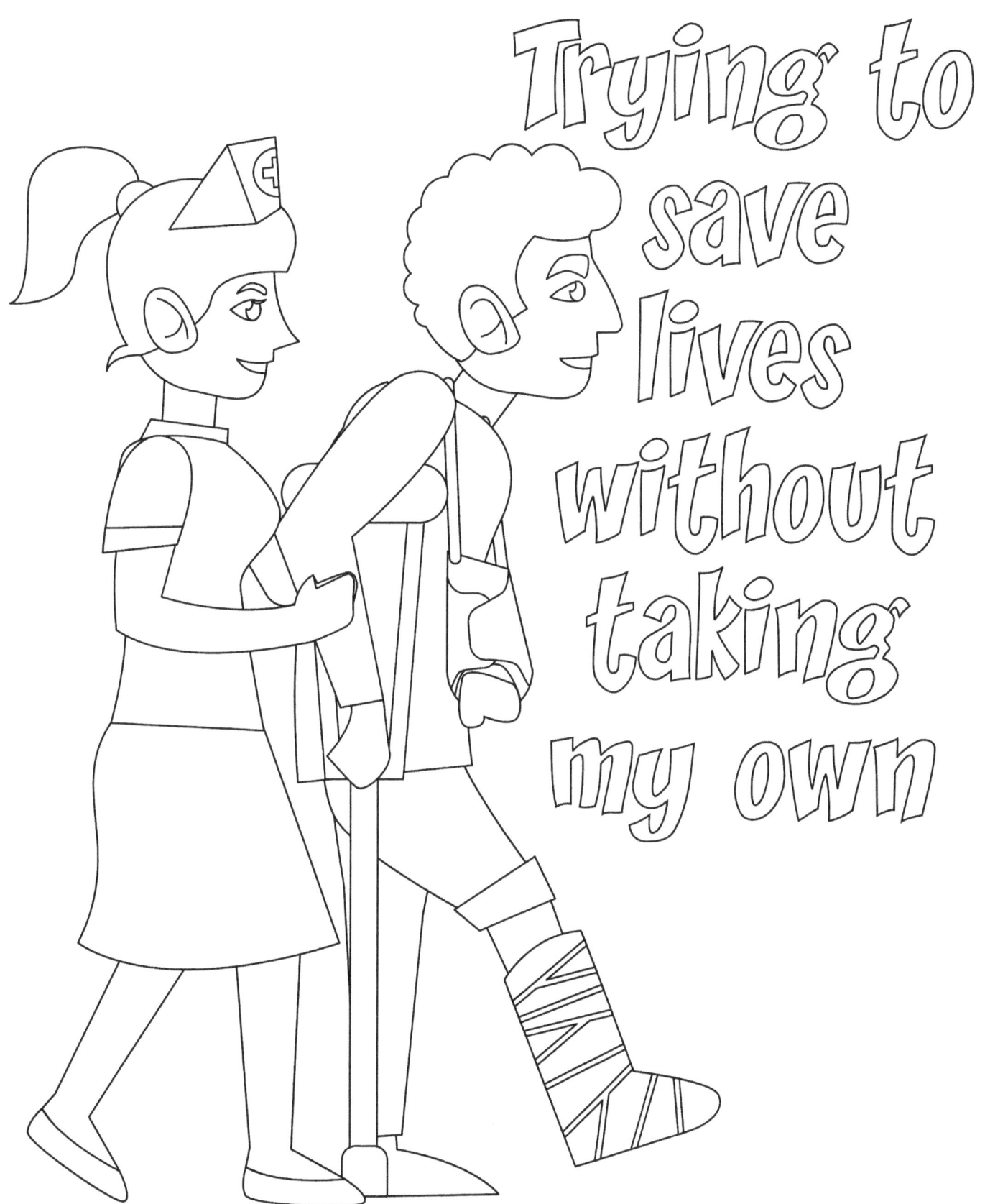

Don't forget to grab your free gift!

https://bit.ly/2K58AtH

Thanks so much for coloring! If you enjoyed this book, please consider leaving a review with what you loved the most ☺ I'm an indie author with no big publishing company or marketing budget behind my projects. Word of mouth and reviews like yours are what help others discover my work! Thank you again for your love and support.

Best,
Megan